PRAISE FOR *THE FATIGUE PRESCRIPTION*

"*The Fatigue Prescription* is a compelling book designed for these busy times; Dr. Clever offers a practical means of taking stock of self, and then embarking on a wise means of renewal."

—Abraham Verghese, author of *Cutting for Stone*

"If you are tired of the army of health experts and their bewilderingly complex, ever-changing advice, *The Fatigue Prescription* is for you. In this practical, crystal-clear book, Dr. Linda Hawes Clever maps a solid plan that will increase your zest and fulfillment in life."

—Larry Dossey, MD, author of *The Power of Premonitions*

"This timely and insightful book is a 'how-to' on maintaining excellence in a helter-skelter world. Dr. Clever—longtime physician at San Francisco's California Pacific Medical Center, a clinical professor at UCSF, and a high-level volunteer (Stanford trustee, KQED board chair)—knows what it's like to have many balls in the air and keep her eye on them all. She shows us how to get back in touch with our basic values and organize our lives around them."

—Elaine Petrocelli, President of Book Passage and www.bookpassage.com

"Linda Hawes Clever, wise physician of the body and of the spirit, has long been an admired national leader in helping others help themselves. In *The Fatigue Prescription,* Dr. Clever has extended her healer's reach to those of us with full, hectic schedules and seemingly not enough energy to deal with them. Drawing upon her extensive experience in the area of renewal, she offers valuable insights for diagnosing and dealing with the fatigue of 'too much to do.' 'Taking care of yourself is not selfish, it's self-preservation' is Dr. Clever's clear and saving message. Here is a prescription worth filling."

—Charles J. Hatem, MD, Harold Amos Academy Professor of Medicine at Harvard Medical School

"Fatigue is the number one problem that I see in my busy psychiatric practice. Women are especially vulnerable. We do too much and yet we have much more to do. Traditional medications don't work, counseling doesn't usually address this problem, and our families and employers always seem to want *more.* Dr. Linda Hawes Clever gives us realistic and practical tools to help all of us live a calmer, more satisfying life. I strongly recommend reading this book as you begin your journey of renewal."

—Leslie Lundt, MD, XM radio host

"This dynamo of a book by renowned physician Dr. Linda Hawes Clever is direct from her heart to yours. This is a one-stop resource for deepening your self-awareness and reconnecting with sources of energy and optimism you may have presumed lost. Just as she promises, you will emerge from this reading experience wiser, happier, healthier!"
—Janet Bickel, MA, career and leadership development coach and consultant

"Fatigue is becoming an American epidemic—and it costs us dearly in personal energy and in our capacity for national progress. In *The Fatigue Prescription*, Linda Hawes Clever, MD, a physician with deep public health experience, supplies wise advice on prevention—and also on recovery and renewal."
—Donald Kennedy, President Emeritus of Stanford University and former editor of *Science*

"'Tired all the time' is named TATT by physicians and is one of the commonest reasons that people consult a physician. This marvelously and lightly written book can help you avoid developing TATT and lead you to a place where being is more important than doing. The time is ripe for all of us to move on from our world of excess and Linda Hawes Clever provides a clear path."
—Richard Smith, MD, former editor of the *British Medical Journal*

"Linda Hawes Clever is a remarkable woman and has written an equally remarkable book to help us all overcome stress, give us the energy to achieve our own best objectives, and rediscover the joy in our lives."
—Arlene Blum, author of *Breaking Trail: A Climbing Life* and Executive Director of the Green Science Policy Institute

"How come many of us are so tired? Does fatigue serve a survival purpose, and if so, what might that purpose be? The antenna of fatigue says, 'Slow down. Rest.' As a back of the pack marathoner for over forty years, I should be a world expert on fatigue, but I am not. Is it muscle lactic acid buildup? Or is it brain fatigue, the cortical cells depleted of staying power? Or is it the spirit that flags in its resolve, looking elsewhere for renewal and respite? Linda Hawes Clever's handsome book takes on these big-issue considerations and helps find resolution to universal fatigue. Read and renew."
—Walter M. Bortz, II, MD, author of *We Live Too Short and Die Too Long* and *Next Medicine*

"If you want a boost to your energy, take Dr. Clever's Renew-O-Meter. Feel the relief, feel renewed. Finally, a book of practical, healthy tips that can be easily taken in daily doses!"
—Jan Yanehiro, Emmy-winning broadcaster

"How do we get through our to-do list day in and day out without getting flat out exhausted? Sounds like a tall order, but *The Fatigue Prescription* gives you concrete strategies to rise above your busy schedule and rediscover the meaning behind the madness. Going beyond quick fixes takes courage and discipline on your part, but this book is packed with easy-to-use interactive tools to bring the vitality and joy back into your life."
—Jamie Woolf, author of *Mom-in-Chief: How Wisdom From the Workplace Can Save Your Family From Chaos*

"How did our lives become so extraordinarily complex? With uncommon insight, Dr. Clever helps pare down the non-essentials and provides a simple four-step prescription to a better life. This book is truly a 'refreshing oasis' from which we can refuel our spirits."
—Eliza Lo Chin, MD, MPH, President-Elect of the American Medical Women's Association and editor of *This Side of Doctoring: Reflections from Women in Medicine*

"People who are too busy—whose only complaint is that the day is not long enough or whose excuse for forgetting things is that their neuron synapses are on overload—are people just like me. The good news is we are often doing just what we want to do and would not want it any other way. But the other side of the story is that often we are so overloaded that fatigue sets in...a level of fatigue that can't be relieved just by a good night's sleep. We are the ones who need *The Fatigue Prescription*. We need this to take control of our lives, rather than feeling that our lives are controlling us. We need to know new rules to work within. Dr. Linda Hawes Clever, in *The Fatigue Prescription,* has given us the new rules...so that we can continue our busy productive lives, but with control.

As nurses, we need to also take time for renewal—personally and professionally. Nurses give so much of themselves to their patients and patients' families in their critical caring role. In order to continue the giving, there needs to be replenishment. Dr. Clever, through years of conversations with nurses, knows this better than we do ourselves. *The Fatigue Prescription* provides us with a pathway for our personal and professional renewal. Without this renewal, fatigue slips in as constant giving without replenishing becomes so wearing that we begin to lose our caring touch. *The Fatigue Prescription* has something in it for every nurse—and for anyone who needs to take control of their busy, over-committed lives."

—Deloras Jones, RN, MS, Executive Director of California Institute for Nursing & Health Care

"In Dr. Clever's extraordinary book, I have found the prescription I need to continue to pursue my life path with purpose and passion, but in good health with minimal workaholic stress. I am sure her wise and broad-based advice will prove a blessing to readers from a host of varied backgrounds, not just overly future-oriented folks like me."

—Philip Zimbardo, PhD, author of *The Time Paradox* and *The Lucifer Effect,* professor emeritus at Stanford University, and professor at the Pacific Graduate School of Psychology

"The renewal process needs constant watering. Linda Hawes Clever has written a great and helpful book that deservedly belongs next to John Gardner's *Self-Renewal. The Fatigue Prescription* is a deep and practical book that will do a world of good for anyone who reads it. It can help all of us learn to go slow in a fast world."

—Jim Thompson, founder of Positive Coaching Alliance

THE
FATIGUE
PRESCRIPTION

THE
FATIGUE
PRESCRIPTION

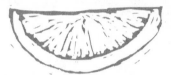

FOUR STEPS TO RENEWING YOUR
ENERGY, HEALTH AND LIFE

LINDA HAWES CLEVER, MD
FOUNDER, RENEW
CLINICAL PROFESSOR OF MEDICINE,
UNIVERSITY OF CALIFORNIA SAN FRANCISCO

V!VA
EDITIONS

Published in the United States by Viva Editions, an imprint of Cleis Press Inc., 2246 Sixth St., Berkeley, California 94710.

Printed in the United States.
Cover design: Scott Idleman
Cover photograph: Image Source
Text design: Frank Wiedemann
First Edition.
10 9 8 7 6 5 4 3 2 1

Grateful acknowledgement is made to the following for granting permission to reprint copyrighted material:

Wendell Berry, "What We Need is Here" from *The Selected Poems of Wendell Berry*. © 1999 by Counterpoint. Reprinted by permission of Counterpoint. C.P. Cavafy "Ithaca" from *The Complete Poems of Cafavy*. English translation copyright © 1961 and renewed 1989 by Rae Dalven, reprinted by permission of Houghton Mifflin Harcourt Publishing Company. UK and Commonwealth reprint rights: "Ithaca" from *The Complete Poems of C.P. Cavafy*, translated by Rae Dalven, published by Chatto & Windus. Reprinted by permission of The Random House Group Ltd. Rev. Forrest Church, excerpt from *Love and Death: My Journey Through the Valley of the Shadow*. © 2008 by the permission of Beacon Press. Langston Hughes, "Dreams" from *The Collected Poems of Langston Hughes*. © 1994 by the Estate of Langston Hughes. Reprinted by permission of Alfred A. Knopf, a division of Random House, Inc. Lao Tzu, "Always We Hope," from *The Way of Life According to Lao Tzu*, translated by Witter Bynner. © 1986 by Harper Collins. Reprinted with permission from Perigee Books. Rumi, "Guest House," from *The Essential Rumi*. © 1997 by HarperOne. Reprinted by permission of Coleman Barks.

Library of Congress Cataloging-in-Publication Data

Clever, Linda Hawes.
 The fatigue prescription : four steps to renewing your energy, health and life / Linda Hawes Clever.
-- 1st ed.
    p. cm.
ISBN 978-1-57344-380-7 (trade paper : alk. paper)
1. Fatigue. 2. Stress management. 3. Self-care, Health. I. Title.
QP421.C54 2010
612.7'44--dc22
                        2009048559

Dedicated to those who tried and try so hard:

My family

ACKNOWLEDGEMENTS

This book has been a lifetime in the works. Aren't all books like that? I watched my mother—an author and teacher of authors—as she toiled, and I thought, "That is way too hard. I want to be a doctor." My life as a wife, mother, and physician, accelerated by more than a decade of renewing and a year of full-court pressing, got me to this point.

Thank you to my parents, Evelyn Johnson Hawes and Nat H. Hawes, who, with my grandparents and teachers from elementary through medical school, gave me unfailing encouragement and generous spirits. My father had remarkable abilities to bring people together and to goad them to unprecedented heights (including the roof of a historic hotel, as he spearheaded renovation work). His resilience and his courage to stand up to opposition were forti-fied by his teasing sense of humor. My mother was more reflec-tive and suffered the way creative people do, especially women in the mid-twentieth century. She, too, was very funny and strong of character. She braved censure by persevering and speaking up with tact and alternatives. Both had remarkable coteries of friends and colleagues. This foundation led eventually and indirectly to this book. Discouragement may have come my way, but I am blessed by their strengths and sense of humor and by a good, albeit short, memory, so obstacles didn't deter.

My husband Jamie, our daughter Sarah, and our son-in-law Keith Gayler have bolstered and cheered me with their advice and gentle inquiries. Their quick responses and forbearance are both comforts and stimuli. Jamie gets the award for supporting "activities of daily living," whether as dish- and clothes-washer or telephone answerer, all while practicing medicine and serving on community boards. I treasure his steady, loving, brown-eyed gaze.

John W. Gardner was instigator, inspiration, and mentor. I greatly value his philosophy, writings, wit, and our innumerable conversations. Other family, friends, acquaintances, and our Community Church have always been there too—sometimes bewildered or amused, but there. I am touched and amazed by the depth and constancy of their caring and kindness. Many have made practical comments, such as poet Margaret Kaufman's "One platitude goes a long way."

Harnessing his empathy and vision, Peter Barnes established Mesa Refuge, a secluded country establishment for writers with special interests. My residency there gave me a delicious, quiet island of time. I cannot imagine being able to formulate and outline this book without living at the sanctuary that edges breathtaking, historic land, marsh, and bay.

A nearby restaurant sports a sign on its door: CRITICS ARE NOT WELCOME. But every author needs them. Over a period of some years, good souls have been willing to read and critique many versions and excerpts of *The Fatigue Prescription*. They have commented with constructive clarity. This hardy band includes Beth Ashley; Marvin Chaney, PhD; David Hill; Robert Rodvien,

MD; and Joan Schretlen. Alev Croutier and members of her writers' salon provided a stimulating, safe, rich milieu and always-useful reviews. Special notice goes to Annie-May De Bresson for being so insistent, and to Mandy Behbehani who, along with Alev, stayed the course through years of rewrites, long after my part in the sessions ended. Classmates Paola Gianturco and Terrell Dougan gave priceless writing and publishing tips. Helen Bing and my agent, calm and elegant Sarah Jane Freymann, have believed in the book since they first saw the manuscript, as has Viva Editions' Brenda Knight. Susanna Margolis and Caroline Pincus made pitch-perfect edits too. I put Susanna through some particularly trying moments, but her classical education, intelligence, and chuckle rescued me time and again. I cannot believe the number of revisions that transcriber-designer Susan Gorski processed, but we both went through reams of paper and cartons of office equipment. Always constructive and willing, Susan has the patience of Job and could have deciphered the Rosetta Stone in two weeks.

Many remarkable people have been deeply involved in developing RENEW's concepts and footprint. "The Big Four"—early RENEW staff members Keven Chriss, Kathleen Clark, Shirley Kelley, and Mary Wade—along with the RENEW Board of Directors: Jan Boller, RN, PhD; Eliza Chin, MD; L. William Eichhorn, MDiv; Gail Glasser; Kathryn Johnson; Amanda Spivey; Kenneth Taymor, JD; Emeritus Directors, Phillp R.Lee, MD and Linda deMello; and the Panel of Advisors: Janet Bickel, MA; Patricia Buffler, PhD, MPH; Robert Beck, MS; Roger Bulger, MD; Kathleen Cardinal; Lisa Chamberlain, MD; Harvey Cohen, MD, PhD; Gretchen de Baubigny; Ann Eichhorn, MDiv, RN; William Foege, MD; Patricia Hellman Gibbs, MD; Laurance Hoagland, MBA; Eric Larson, MD; Iris Litt, MD; Michael Roosevelt, Esq; Bruce Spivey, MD; Marshall Turner, MS, MBA; and Mary Woolley, MA. Program coordinator

Keven Chriss, in particular, has served RENEW as communications hub, glue, and energizer for years. Well supplied with good sense, an infectious laugh, and a willingness to try anything that is reasonable, she is devoted and intrepid.

Finally, thousands of people across the land support RENEW with gusto. They provide ideas, stories, and links. I respect and cherish them all, which is why they are so well represented in *The Fatigue Prescription*.

As my mother used to say, "I wish it could be diamonds and rubies." But it can't be. I would, however, like to express my deepest gratitude to all of the Encouragers named here, in the book, and in my heart. Thank you. Thank you.

CONTENTS

FOREWORD

Like many people, it's a continual struggle for me to find the right balance between doing good work in the world and enjoying my life. The irony was not lost on me many years ago when I locked myself in a room to finish writing a book, *Love & Survival*, about the healing power of love and community... The book was overdue; they're not called "dead-lines" for nothing.

Ultimately, I realized that this is a false choice. When I take care of myself, I can be much more useful in the world. You can't give what you don't have. The first organ that your heart pumps blood to is itself so that it can then take care of the rest of your body. And if your heart fails to nurture itself, your survival is impaired.

Dr. Linda Hawes Clever knows this from her own experience. She was inspired to write *The Fatigue Prescription* because of her own hard-won wisdom. Dr. Clever's life experience emboldened her to help others avoid fatigue and the hardships that accompany it. "Physician, heal thyself" and she did.

Now, she is sharing her unique knowledge with you in this book. The timing is perfect, as we now live in a world that demands so much of us. She offers the science of self-help and practical, profound, and proven methods for wellness.

The Fatigue Prescription is remarkable because it uses facts, stories, and important questions to encourage readers to dig deeper and live a life authentic to their own values. What you eat, how you respond to stress, and the quality of your relationships and social support may be as powerful as drugs and surgery in avoiding and treating many chronic diseases and fatigue. Readers who take Dr. Clever's good prescription and excellent advice will find they are healthier, calmer, and happier, and have a new lease on life.

Dean Ornish, MD
Founder and President of the Preventive Medicine Research Institute (www.pmri.org)
Clinical Professor of Medicine at the University of California, San Francisco
Author of *The Spectrum*

INTRODUCTION

Tired? Feeling pressed and underappreciated? Low on energy? Grumpy? *Often* grumpy? Sighing a lot? Headachy? Backachy? Losing your creative edge? *On* the edge? Calendar more of a wishlist than a schedule?

You are not alone. And this book is for you. It will show you how to get beyond fatigue.

I have spent years as a multitasking physician. I've tried to be a good wife, parent, speaker, counselor, and community volunteer while working to prevent people from getting sick or injured. I tried to heal them when prevention didn't work. I've seen people get sicker and more tired despite my best efforts and theirs. I have come to realize that, along with hazards, habits, and jobs, the lives of most of the people around us demand almost too much of us.

I didn't think much about overdoing it except to apply bandages to patients and friends—until the wheels fell off of my own life. In one eighteen-month period, my parents died, our house was burglarized, I lost two jobs, and my husband Jamie was diagnosed with cancer. One ray of light was our daughter Sarah. My spirits went from flying high to sinking forty thousand leagues under the sea. Not only was I devastated and overwhelmed, I was *tired.*

Many devoted, capable people with plenty of good things going on and lots to look forward to are felled by fatigue. My fatigue came from too much sorrow. Yours may, too. Or from overreaching and overworking. Or all of the above. You long to do more for your family, your work, and the world, yet you can't get up the steam to get going; you're just too darned tired. The dangerous endpoint is to shut down.

After months of mourning and hoping, it became clear to me that the people and structures I had counted on had vanished. I saw that I needed to renew, refresh, and rebuild my whole life. When I was finally able to look around, I also saw that too many other people were suffering. Some had losses; others had anxieties and uncertainties. Most were soldiering on with huge loads of work and responsibilities, no longer bright-eyed and bushy-tailed. Some wondered if they could keep on at their pace without losing their zest; Something had to be done. There had to be a better way.

My good friend and mentor, John W. Gardner, former Secretary of the Unites States Department of Health, Education and Welfare and founder of Common Cause, had written on leadership, excellence, and renewing. I decided this was the time to put John's theory of renewing into practice. But how?

First I revisited the values that underlay my commitments and therefore my calendar. The things that matter most to me include family, friends, and wanting to make a difference through medicine. Early on, I didn't know how to get beyond re-certifying my values, but with John's advice and prodding, I started to give talks at meetings and seminars for doctors, nurses, teachers, volunteers, churchgoers, executives, and other leaders. I asked questions and listened as people attested to the importance of renewing. Then I asked them to list the ways they did it. I kept track of all the answers. As ideas crystallized, some friends and I organized the not-for-profit RENEW. John gave a rousing keynote speech at our first one-and-a-half-day gathering. He pointed out that meaning is something you build into your life. The link between finding meaning in your life and conquering fatigue is to renew yourself—your spirit, energy, dreams, and relationships. Paying attention to others and myself, I took on a do-it-yourself project to do just that.

Over the decade since starting RENEW, I have determined that most of us go through four steps to restore ourselves. It isn't a direct path from the first to the last step, either. You may well meander, take a rest, double back, or detour. That's all right, because you have a tested, successful approach to guide you. This approach has worked for thousands—including me—and I believe it will work for you. I call it the Fatigue Prescription.

Perhaps because I am a physician, I have faith in prescriptions—the right ones taken at the right times. *The Fatigue Prescription: Four Steps to Renewing Your Energy, Health and Life* shows how to maintain or regain the passion, the warmth, the vigor—and the results, accomplishments, and successes—you seek. Its step-by-step formula will show you how to discover your own remedies for fatigue so you can overcome the exhaustion that interferes with your life.

I hope many pages in this book will get dog-eared because you use it so much. I hope you will have fun and write all over it, as you tussle with ideas, answer questions, check boxes, and scribble in the margins. The notes you make will reinforce your learning and memory, because when your brain and muscles work together, this neuro-physiological partnership engraves ideas and actions into you. My purpose is to tattoo RENEWing and the Fatigue Prescription into your thoughts.

The tried and true Renew-O-Meter is a good starting point. We designed it to help jugglers like you gauge your feelings and behavior. Fill in the blanks and begin to think about how pleased you are with your life—or how tired you are. And how you would like your life to be.

THE RENEW-O-METER

Your answers to these questions (one answer per question) will help you measure how deftly you juggle your commitments and how much you could benefit from renewing.

ONE: How many times did you really laugh yesterday?	
0 (0 points)	
1–2 (1 point)	
3–4 (2 points)	
5–6 (3 points)	
7+ (4 points)	
TWO: How often do you learn something new?	
Haven't learned a new subject in the last year (0 points)	
I'm focused exclusively on my field (1 point)	
I read or search widely beyond my field (2 points)	
I take courses outside my field (3 points)	
I teach others (4 points)	

THREE: How many times in the past three days do you (or others) think you overreacted, let a little thing get to you in a big way?	
0 (4 points)	
1–2 (3 points)	
3–4 (2 points)	
5–6 (1 point)	
7+ (0 points)	

FOUR: How often in the past month did you feel trapped, a prisoner of circumstances?	
Never (4 points)	
Once or twice (3 points)	
Three or four times (2 points)	
Five or six times (1 point)	
More than seven times (0 points)	

FIVE: How often do you typically have conversations with friends outside of your profession?	
Every day or two (4 points)	
Once a week (3 points)	
Every other week (2 points)	
Once a month (1 point)	
A few times a year (0 points)	

SIX: When did you last feel bold enough to take a risk?	
Within the past week (4 points)	
1–2 weeks ago (3 points)	
3–8 weeks ago (2 points)	
3–6 months ago (1 point)	
Can't remember (0 points)	

SEVEN: How many sit-down dinners did you have with your family or friends in the past week?	
0 (0 points)	
1–2 (1 point)	
3–4 (2 points)	
5–6 (3 points)	
7+ (4 points)	

EIGHT: How many times in the past week did you spend more than one hour refreshing your body or spirit (not counting eating or sleeping)?	
6+ (4 points)	
4–5 (3 points)	
2–3 (2 points)	
1 (1 point)	
None (0 points)	

NINE: How often do consider your own aspirations when you make decisions?	
My what? (0 points)	
Rarely (1 point)	
Sometimes (2 points)	
Frequently (3 points)	
Always (4 points)	

TEN: When was the last time you encouraged someone?	
Today (4 points)	
This week (3 points)	
This month (2 points)	
Two or three months ago (1 point)	
Six months ago or more (0 points)	
Your Score =	

Score	Diagnosis
31 – 40	Superstar juggler. You're doing great. Keep renewing your*self* and others.
25 – 30	All-star juggler. You have plenty of balls in the air, but you're paying a price. What will you do to renew?
20 – 24	Two-star juggler. You're probably worried about how you will keep all those balls in the air. This is a splendid time to reflect and renew.
0 – 19	No-star juggler. You seem to have too many balls in the air, or you could be discouraged or overwhelmed. Think about making a quick U-turn toward renewing!

PART ONE

THE DIAGNOSIS

CHAPTER 1

HOW DID YOU GET SO BUSY? HOW DID YOU GET SO TIRED?

I arise...torn between a desire to improve the world and a desire to enjoy the world. This makes it hard to plan the day.

—E.B. White

No wonder you're tired! You have wants and needs. You want to get a lot done and you want to do it well. Your family and friends need and expect your attention. So does your checkbook. You also have plenty of *should*s and *ought to*s. You *should* be an informed voter. You *ought* to get some exercise. And for goodness sake, you want to see a good movie sometime soon! In your rare quiet times, you realize that you want to be better than busy. You want some time to think and plan. You want some peace and quiet without feeling guilty and selfish.

This book puts your closest buddy—you—into the driver's seat, moving out of the rat race and into fatigue-free good health.

How?

In medicine, we try to determine the cause of the symptoms—

the diagnosis—and then we can design the appropriate treatment: the remedy. That is what I hope this book does for you.

In this chapter, you and I will sort out the whys and wherefores—some of the reasons you have accumulated so many demands and commitments, what these relentless responsibilities are, and what they may be doing to you. You'll give your energy bucket the once-over and come up with a couple of favors you can do for yourself. After discussing two important qualities—courage and pride—the chapter wraps up with a preview of the Fatigue Prescription and its four steps.

Later in Part One, since this is the diagnosis section, you'll do your own checkup and see the Prescription's benefits. Soon you'll be well positioned to launch into the remedy. Part Two, The Renewing Remedy, uses the Prescription's four steps to help you reconnect with your values and discover what you really want and how to get it. You'll see how others have renewed their bodies, spirits, and energy. You will get some quick tips and ideas for long-term maintenance.

Why all this emphasis on *you*? Because you are important! And it is not selfish to take care of yourself. It is self-preservation so you can do what you want to do or must do. *You* are the one who can best take care of yourself. No one else can do it as well, and no one else cares about you as much.

By way of example, and to help you start understanding the challenges you may face and the way you may approach them—and why—let me tell you about a young musician. She was trying to make a living by patching together jobs as a church choir director, a high-school rehearsal accompanist, a greeting card designer, and a piano teacher—all while she was thinking about a new career, hunting for a full-time job, dealing with family demands, and dating an interesting guy. One day she came home to find her low-rent apartment flooded with sewage. The manager said he would fix the drainage system, but when the apartment flooded for a second time, her spirits hit bottom. She was angry, and she felt betrayed. She caught a cold, snapped at her friends and students, and cried. Anybody would! She was stuck, however, with no money, a tight schedule, and lots of distractions. She was determined to fix the problem but didn't want to add a disruptive move to her situation. So she enlisted her father's help. He checked the plumbing and made firm recommendations to the manager. She persuaded the manager to pay for the cleanup so she wouldn't have to call the health department. When the dust and goo settled, she had an after-the-flood-get-together. Her grit and network got her through.

Where do you get your grit, and how do you develop your network? What about your drive, even your tastes and preferences? How did you get so much on your plate that you got exhausted and, perhaps worse, stale? Nature, nurture, combinations, circumstances? All of these, most likely.

INCLINATIONS YOU ARE BORN WITH: YOUR INHERITANCE

Parents notice differences in behavior between identical twins on day one—sometimes even in utero! One sucks a thumb while the other does somersaults. Twins or not, birth order and gender alone don't explain why an older brother is placid and the younger sister is zippy. Although it is true that the intrauterine environment and mother's hormones play some part, siblings' very own genetic makeup, the way that chemicals spiral in their DNA, makes a powerful difference.

The reasons why you like strawberry and she likes butterscotch, why one runs fast and another is better on the balance beam, why somebody prefers mysteries and someone else biographies, are mainly innate. Personality traits are affected by rewards and punishments—high grades for being thorough, time-outs for punching another kid in day care—yet we all start with our own basic tendencies.

Those of us who are super busy may choose to be that way for a number of reasons. You may load your schedule because you want approval or to please others. You may set very high standards for yourself. You may want to win or to set a record. Any of these can lead to saying yes to so many requests that your to-do list is long enough to tie into bows. You may be running away. (A fellow told me not long ago, "I'd rather work overtime than deal with my teenager.")

A tendency to overload to the point of fatigue may be part of your inherited package; it may run in your family, just like hair color does. This may seem inconsequential, but it isn't. Fatigue can drain your enthusiasm and effectiveness, and if you've inherited a legacy of fatigue, you could be in a hole from the start. Of course, your inherited traits aren't the whole story. Plenty of external influences affect you as well.

GROWING UP

I could discuss an array of ways that your personality and biochemistry—such as fatigue and hair color— may be trumped or amplified by your habits and surroundings. For example, a good diet and sufficient exercise can help thwart hereditary heart troubles. If your environment isn't conducive to addictive behavior, even if you are prone to addiction, you may have no problem. Depression, which is traceable through generations, may not surface if misfortunes don't strike or if you develop ways to cope. So, too, can fatigue be managed. Although genes can make you more susceptible to fatigue, prevention helps. Which is why you're reading this book!

Expectations are another set of external forces that can push you to cram your calendar. In my view, expectations are, at best, double-edged swords. There is no question that having deadlines and goals is good for motivation. They get your juices flowing, set your eyes on the prize, move you ahead. But the problem comes when you don't set your own expectations, when someone else sets your expectations for you. Who defines what a person's "success" in life will be? I once heard a conversation between two men, both professionals, on that subject. One said that his definition of success was being a CEO. The other said it was "being able to talk to my daughter." Who or what shaped those opinions? Think about it: Who picked which music lessons you took? Which instrument—piano, drums, or ocarina? Which style—jazz, country, or classical? Who had what hopes about what you would accomplish? Are you a neatnik or do you collect dust bunnies? Who decides when it's time to clean your room? Do you watch sports or play sports? Which ones? Who says?

One of the biggest expectations set for you by others can be your choice of work or profession. How many stories have you heard—or lived—about people who followed their parents' desires rather than their own? This could push you into the family restaurant or auto repair business, or could send you on the path to being a lawyer or a politician. It's one thing when you have an epiphany, an *aha!* or a calling. In that case, you eagerly channel your energy and intentions in a certain direction because they represent your own desires. But it's another matter when you are walking in anothers' shoes because someone *expect*s you to do so. Those shoes can be hard to fill, and are often harder to lift with each step. That is exhausting!

I admire my cousin, Steve Hawes, for many reasons, not only because he had a ten-year career in the NBA. His son Ellis is about

Steve's height and has become a great guitar player. Ellis never had much more than a flicker of interest in basketball, the sport his dad mastered. Thankfully, Steve and Ebs, Ellis' mother, didn't pressure him to become a basketball player. Ellis was drawn in another direction and lives according to his own expectations. His parents are fine with his choice.

Sometimes, the expectations can be a *folie à deux*, a condition in which the symptom or delusion of one person is transferred to another. I recall a physician whose physician father had an unerring instinct that he applied to diagnostic challenges. The younger doctor admired that skill enormously, and his father wanted him to be his partner in practice. The young man plodded through medical school and residency, doing well enough. It took several years for both men to realize that the younger doctor's interests were in administration, not clinical practice. He now uses his background and his passion at the helm of a leading hospital.

YOUR ENERGY BUCKET

Let's face it. You have a lot to do. You are magnetic. You take on countless pleasures and obligations that mesh with your genetic inclinations and upbringing. This adds up to having a lot on your mind that can deplete your energy.

Here are some items that people across the country report are on their minds and that require mental energy. Part of dealing with fatigue is recognizing what's out there—or *in* there—taking up space in your mind. Look over the list and circle your own stuff that is weighing on you.

STUFF ON MY MIND	
Work	Coworkers
Family	Two jobs
The economy	Lovers
Kids	My expectations of me versus others' expectations of me
Commute	Child going into the Marines
Money	Having fun
Friends	Making time for myself
Sleep	School
Hobbies	My wife's parents and my father are both sick and live far from us
Housekeeping	My health—mental and physical
Professional organizations	Politics
House guests	Learning something new
Deadlines	...*plus* my other stuff
Education	

To add to things that are already on your mind, you may be cruising along, eyes bright, wind in your hair, exhilarated with your feats, when *BOOM*, more stuff happens. Small episodes can derail you. Think about a fender bender, a head cold, or my friend's sewage episodes. Your body could let you down with illness, injury, or nutritional and hormonal insufficiencies. A divorce or death, losing an election, a job, or sleep, even much-anticipated retirement can deplete your energy. Your usual support systems and feelings of capability evaporate into uncertainty. To top it all off, unsettling events tend to cluster. My mother used to say, "Sometimes you have a bad *year*." You have good ones, too, but may not notice that. At any rate, fatigue can become a companion when circumstances gang up.

When bad things happen to good, busy people, your body, emotions, memory, relationships, and work feel it. A while back, I asked a group of new medical students about their feelings when pressures build up and they get tired. It took no time at all for them to come up with this list:

MEDICAL STUDENTS' SIGNS OF TROUBLE	
Get sick—catch cold, etc.	Apathy
Lose patience	Restlessness
Stop caring	Stop hanging out with friends
Stop reflecting	Denial
Stop sleeping	Crying
Decreased appetite	Hostility
Stop eating	Impatience
Start eating	Irritability
Cranky	Just walk around pissed off

Now list your own signs of trouble. Include physical symptoms, feelings, intellectual reactions, energy level, and the effects on your relationships, job, and anything else you've observed.

MY SIGNS OF TROUBLE

Diana Arsham, a psychologist and a walking buddy of mine, points out that each of us has an energy bucket:

You may start out with your bucket quite full or mostly empty, depending upon your inheritance, experiences, and situations. But regardless of where the level starts, it is important to check it on a regular basis, especially when demands are high. There are many things that could cause your energy bucket to leak: health, duties, arguments, expectations, and so forth. The idea is to:

- Determine where the holes are
- Plug them with "corks"
- Add new energy

The "corks" that plug the holes may include going to the doctor, getting counseling, or recruiting help with your household chores. You might say "No" more often, send out for more Chinese food, or make a tough decision and stick with it. The new energy may come in many forms as well. Short boosts could come from going for a walk, writing in a journal, or taking a power nap with the office door shut. You might sing (just about anywhere), play with a child, play catch with Rover, or talk to a friend on the phone. Longer-term fixes may stem from adjusting schedules, attitudes, or interactions, or curbing those late nights on weekdays—or weekends.

It is useful to know what does it every time for you, what always lifts you up. So take a deep breath, let your shoulders relax from up around your ears, and make a list right on this page:

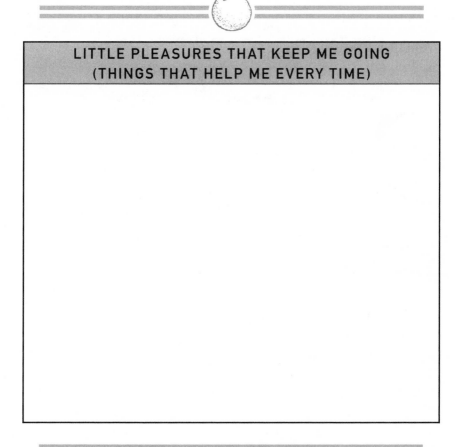

**LITTLE PLEASURES THAT KEEP ME GOING
(THINGS THAT HELP ME EVERY TIME)**

Since you are thinking about energy bucket maintenance, take this chance to look at some routine ways to keep your level high. The following chart offers some food for thought. All of these activities take some time. That's okay! You can make the time. You might want to add other pursuits that are important to you and adapt the chart to fit your preferred timing. Renewing your energy bucket, just like exercise, needs to be a regular part of your life, not a sporadic add-on or an emergency "must."

SOME GOOD WAYS TO MAINTAIN A FULL ENERGY BUCKET

EVERY DAY
Get up, get washed and dressed
Stretch
Clean up your room / apartment / house
Eat well
Follow recommendations to maintain or regain health
Have some fun
Work (for pay or not)
Connect with family and friends
Take care of pets
Read a book or magazine or blog
Sleep
Study current events
Smile, laugh
Accomplish something
Thank someone
My ways:

EVERY WEEK
Do laundry
Take out the trash
Pay your bills
Go grocery shopping
Garden, indoors or outdoors
Indulge (within reason)
My ways:

EVERY MONTH
Balance checkbook
Experience "culture"
Go out to eat
Attend or organize a community meeting
Get a haircut
Buy a toy or book or puzzle
Watch a funny movie
My ways:

EVERY THREE MONTHS
Take a mini vacation at a favorite or new place
Recycle, organize your files, or toss clutter
Fulfill a dream
Get a gadget
Play
My ways:

EVERY YEAR
Take a maxi vacation
Get health check and immunizations
Pay your taxes
Vote
Celebrate holidays
Kick back
My ways:

COURAGE AND PRIDE

The way you react is a combination of your intrinsic character-istics—how well you see and hear, your tolerance of order or disorder, your capacity for change—plus outside upbringing, traditions, experience, and demands.

Courage and pride rank among the most mysterious and important qualities we humans have. Their genesis is unclear and complicated, although both have to do with values, those basic principles that can get you through tough spots. The bad news is that fatigue can erode even your most cherished beliefs and qualities. A rocky night's sleep can turn a doting grandpa into a grouch.

Courage, which I'll consider first, comes in different forms. Poet Mary Anne Radmacher-Hershey wrote: "Courage doesn't always roar. Sometimes it's the quiet voice at the end of the day saying, 'I will try again tomorrow.'" Firefighters and neighbors rescue people from burning buildings. Activists march. Kids face up to bullies. Reporters ask probing questions. Patients take on another round of chemotherapy.

The ability to take a stand or take a risk springs from our center—at least that's what the Romans thought. "Courage" is derived from *cor*, Latin for "heart." When you take something to heart, when it matters most to you, you can be brave, persist, defy. You can hold true. You can hold hands.

Our daughter Sarah was four years old when she and I gathered with friends at the finish line of the Dipsea Race, a grueling 6.7-mile cross-country run that courses up hundreds of steps and down treacherous trails. My husband Jamie hoped to be in the forefront. As we craned to see, we soon heard gasps and exclamations: "Oh no!" "Look at his face!" "Oh my God!" It was Jamie. He had fallen near the end of the race and impaled his cheek on a jagged rock. He knew he needed medical care, and the only way to get it was to keep on running with a chunk of flesh hanging from his face. We met Jamie at the finish line, piled into the car, and headed to Marin General Hospital, where doctors saw him immediately. I headed off to fill out forms while Sarah stayed with Jamie. When I caught up with them, he was pale, lying on the emergency room gurney, and she was standing close to him, holding his hand. She looked at me and said, "Now, Mommy, would you please hold my hand?" She had stood by, sustaining her dear father despite her terror. Love is a value that provides courage.

Courage can roar, too. In wartime, it roars every day. Signing up and then showing up for duty are plucky in themselves. Battle can ratchet *pluck* up to *valor*. When soldiers live to tell why they pulled a wounded comrade out of the line of fire or threw themselves on live ammunition, their answers are often along the lines of, "I did it for my buddies." That's loyalty and love at work. When Lali Thambiaiyah was a young physician in her homeland, Sri Lanka, her responsibilities included visiting a refugee camp. While she was at the camp, her hospital, three miles away, was attacked. Sixty-eight patients, doctors, nurses, and neighbors were massacred, including her mother-in-law. She went back to the hospital as soon as the shelling stopped, walking past bodies sprawled along the roadside. That's dedication and love at work.

Giving *pride* its due: a little pride can help you go a long way. Wanting to keep your pride makes you prepare like crazy—put a sparkle in your eye, lift up your chin, and straighten your shoulders before you wade into a roomful of strangers. It may be an act, but you feel brighter. That is the way others see you, too. However inborn or trained it is, pride can help you push forward or even survive. I am reminded of one of the physicians whom I admired the most. He was a hero to his patients and had helped found and preside over several national medical associations. He was well into his eighties when his eyesight failed, his pancreas gave out, and he broke his arm. His life already was much circumscribed by difficulty walking. We were close enough that I could ask in conversation, "Have you considered committing suicide?" He said, "Yes." I snapped to full attention and asked, "Do you know how you would do it?" "Yes." "Do you have the means?" "Yes." "Would you go through with it?" He said, "No. I don't want to have it on my record."

But pride can be difficult, too. It can make you vulnerable to criticism and can make you flare or shut down. It can get you stuck. I know a talented young man with three children who is the first in his family to own a business. When the nearby magnet store closed down, his business shrank. He didn't want to cut his losses and go back to school or work for someone else, so he offered new products and cut expenses. He said, "I have my pride." Then the economy got really bad, and he couldn't pay the rent, including, finally, the rent on his own home. He closed shop. Perhaps his pride shouldn't have depended as much on owning his business as on being able to accommodate to change. Charles Darwin said, "In the struggle for survival, the fittest win out at the expense of their rivals because they succeed in adapting themselves best to their environment."

Courage and pride, often coupled with values, can help you make tough choices and persevere. Conquering addiction, for example, takes all of the courage, pride, and values that anyone has, and it often takes help from others, as well. "Addiction" to being on the run and its resultant fatigue can become embedded in you. As far as we know, this addiction does not affect brain biochemistry the way alcohol and nicotine do. All probably share similar causes, however: inheritance, upbringing, and circumstances.

THE FOUR STEPS

The step-by-step Fatigue Prescription will engage you in finding your own remedies to your over-whelm and under-joy. Since you know yourself best and you've gotten this far, you have the solutions. But—with the help of this book—you may need to explore and dig a bit to find them. The effort is well worth your while, for you will make more than life-altering discoveries. They will be life-*saving* discoveries.

The four steps of this prescription are based on my experience and research. Some of the research was at RENEW workshops, listening to thousands of people who wanted to lift up their lives, and thousands more who already have.

The first step is **awareness**. The next is **reflection**. The third is **conversation**. The last is **plan-and-act**. In other words, the way to handle fatigue is to see, think, talk, test, and then do.

AWARENESS
REFLECTION
CONVERSATION
PLAN-AND-ACT

One of the more unique elements of the prescription is its insistence on *conversation*. In your noisy, demanding days, you rarely take the opportunity to chew over brainstorms or to touch base with important people in your life. You lose the savor; you may lose ideas and allies. Safe conversations build resilience and perseverance, two qualities that return when you beat fatigue.

Here is how the prescription works. You begin with **awareness**, or seeing, as you define and describe the nature of your own fatigue. You then **reflect** upon and assemble the resources you have and can deploy—values, people, and dreams. Next you learn how to have important **conversations** with loved ones and colleagues to test your observations and hear others'. Finally, as you move toward **plans and action**, you make some decisions about your purpose and strategy. Along the way, you let go of the chaff and save the wheat. This allows you to clarify what ultimately has worth to you—the meaning in your life. This is an act of transformation and of renewal. It grants you the freedom to make a fresh start.

You can do it. It has been done before.

About 2600 years ago, legendary scholar Lao Tzu captured the hope, the truth, and the remedy for fatigue—and put you in the center.

ALWAYS WE HOPE

Always we hope
someone else has the answer.
Some other place will be better,
some other time it will all turn out.
This is it.
No one else has the answer.
No other place will be better,
and it has already turned out.
At the center of your being
you have the answer;
you know who you are
and you know what you want.
There is no need
to run outside
for better seeing.
Nor to peer from a window.

Rather abide at the center of your being;
for the more you leave it, the less you learn.
Search your heart
and see
the way to do
is to be.

(Translated by Witter Bynner)

The Prescription is not a one-shot deal, of course. Life goes on. The Prescription is meant to be re-filled, just as you need to re-fill your energy bucket and your car. The Prescription shows the way to two victories: sustaining renewal and beating fatigue, twin concepts that I equate.

CHAPTER 2

YOUR OWN CHECKUP

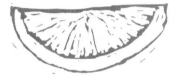

In spite of illness, in spite even of the archenemy sorrow, one can remain alive long past the usual date of disintegration if one is unafraid of change, insatiable in intellectual curiosity, interested in big things, and happy in small ways.

—Edith Wharton

As I left my house the other day, I glanced down the street and saw a neighbor careening toward her car. Her arms were overflowing with loose papers, a brightly striped canvas bag (also overflowing), and workout clothes. Her mouth was full, too, her teeth clenching an insulated coffee mug. I ran to help her open the car door, but she beat me to it. She looked a little wild-eyed and gasped, "I'm so busy!" I could see that. She went on apologetically, "I try to meditate every day. But it's the same ol' same ol'. Shouldn't I be making *progress*?" I said that my computer was down for the third time in a week and my e-mailbox was so full that incoming messages would soon be stopped. "I'm trying to be Zen," I told her. "You know, 'in the moment'. But I don't like the moment!" She told about a bumper sticker that she had just seen: "Life may be short, but it sure is wide."

The kind of fatigue you can feel may be wide and deep. It is the sheer exhaustion that comes when you have done way too much and it doesn't seem to be enough. You may feel like you are in a bottomless pit of requirements and duties.

This isn't burnout. Burnout certainly includes exhaustion, but it is coupled with cynicism and low self-esteem. It is often related to your job (including volunteering) or profession. Burnout worms its way into you when reality overwhelms your expectations and you can no longer tolerate what you are doing. You can't fix what you don't like. You cannot even walk through the office door.

The fatigue I'm describing is different. It doesn't necessarily stop you. It stops your effectiveness and pleasure. It drains your energy and saps your health and your life. That counts.

I am also not describing the kind of fatigue that comes with depression. Depression is a medical condition that can fluctuate for decades, with intense feelings of inadequacy, gloominess, and lethargy. This miasma not only affects emotions, but can infiltrate bodies, including bowel movements. Depression immobilizes so much that a person may stay in bed for days on end, and literally get constipated.

The Fatigue Prescription treats a different kind of fatigue, the fatigue you feel when you get out of bed and survey the landscape of activities and priorities facing you—and realize that you are already tired. Or you wilt at the end of the day or week because you look back and feel like you have not accomplished anything meaningful—and you haven't had a spare minute to send a get-well card or snuggle with the cat, either.

The Fatigue Prescription aims to restore something you once had: excitement and passion about your work, your friends and family, your causes, your life, *yourself.* You miss that groove and those highs. Or you are worried they are trickling away. Be ready to feel the stir, the warmth, the vigor, and the energy you once had—and savor the results. Let's start on your quest.

This chapter has several appraisals for you. They are about vital topics: your feelings, effectiveness, body, spirit, and relationships. After you take these appraisals, I will suggest and expand upon two major determinants of your ability to combat fatigue: your learning and your attitude.

HOW ARE YOU FEELING AND DOING THESE DAYS?

Sometimes, deliberately or not, you pack your days so full you don't have to feel. You may not even be aware that your toothache is getting worse until you try to go to sleep at night. Or that your boss' put down really got under your skin. Busyness can be a great anesthetic, but it is only temporary and doesn't deal with the source of the pain.

The Fatigue Prescription gets back to basics by helping you figure out how you're really feeling. That is how the Prescription starts: with *awareness.*

It's important to be aware of feelings because they do not go away. Fear, anger, boredom, and sorrow may seem to lie dormant but are actually simmering and can explode. I recall a friend who fell in love at the same time that her mother was dying. My friend buried her grief and guilt for a decade, but when her marriage started to fail and the couple sought counseling, her unresolved feelings about her mother surfaced as the primary cause of disputes. Exploring those feelings led to forgiving herself, and the marital tensions eased.

Feelings tend to be complicated. My friend's loss and sadness intertwined with her love and happiness. Sometimes the sadness compounds, as when financial worries accompany illness. Sometimes thrills and difficulties mesh: getting a new job and leaving home, bringing a new baby home to a 650-square-foot apartment, returning from a relaxing break to towers of mail. Emotions and physical conditions can combine, too. A friend who was contending with a divorce, teenagers, and menopause lamented, "Feelings and hormones rule!" It's a mix-and-match world with powerful forces braided together.

Get comfy and check out these questions. You can fill in the blanks or circle the answers and write some comments, or you might just give the page a glance and then stare out the window for a while.

HOW AM I FEELING AND DOING?
Do I have any signs of trouble, such as body aches, flairs of anger, or changes in weight or sleeping habits? ❑ Yes ❑ No
Am I rarin' to go or runnin' on empty? Comment:
Am I grateful or grouchy? Comment:

HOW AM I FEELING AND DOING?
How am I doing with my responsibilities (parents, partner, kids, paying bills, pulling weeds, folding clothes)? Comment:
Have I had fun in the last week or two? ❏ Yes ❏ No If yes, doing what?
Have I learned anything new in the last couple of months (how to fix that infernal faucet; a good new mystery writer; the names of the countries of the former Soviet Union; *any*thing)?
How is my ability to concentrate? ❏ Fine ❏ Dwindling ❏ Say what?
I make very few mistakes (for example, I remember my appointments). ❏ True ❏ False ❏ Don't bug me
What's the trend? Are my signs of trouble ❏ Increasing? ❏ Decreasing? ❏ Staying about the same?

Mull over your answers and see if they raise your awareness about how you are feeling or doing these days. This is the first step toward dissipating your fatigue.

BODY BEAUTIFUL (OR AT LEAST BODY HEALTHY)

This checklist is not about mere appearances. It is about having a healthy body. Good physical health is probably the best fuel for your energy bucket. Diminished health—from pain, worry, illness, and so forth—makes you tired. Of course, it is possible to triumph over these impediments. Franklin Delano Roosevelt was a brilliant strategist despite polio; Helen Keller learned to communicate despite being deaf and blind; my mother published, taught, and mothered beautifully despite crippling migraines. But it is better to prevent or alleviate the problem—and the fatigue. This is why I offer some facts and measurements, along with recommendations about good health and good health practices.

These guidelines aren't forever because knowledge and science march on. The guidelines do not fit everyone perfectly because everyone has a specific heredity and environment. The checklist is a reasonable start to maintaining your body as well as you can, however. This is fundamental to conquering the loss of function and the fatigue that can accompany being below par.

Your checkup need not be frequent or fancy. It is just a routine part of having a full energy bucket and a robust life. The whole megillah will take maybe half a day per year.

First of all, find a "medical home," a health professional who listens carefully, is well–informed, and works in a system that meets your needs. One clue to the first criterion is that she/he is quiet for more than twenty seconds without interrupting your narrative. Clues to the second point include the clinician's attending professional meetings, reading professional journals, being board-certified and re-certified, and perhaps being on a medical school part-time or full-time faculty. You should be sure that your practitioner is free of disciplinary actions, so check your state medical board's Web site.

Where can you find this paragon if you don't already have one? The search is especially challenging because primary-care practitioners for adults are in short supply. Go beyond the advice from family and friends. Keep trying! Your search for excellence may lead you to the most distinguished nearby hospital's medical staff office or residency training program, or to a medical school. Find out where their chief residents from the last ten to fifteen years have gone into practice. Your local or regional medical society could also be a good source. With whomever you find, you may want to arrange a trial appointment that you pay for.

Your first-rate clinician not only needs to be smart, but also available. Of course, doctors must have time to renew and restore themselves so they can take good care of you. When they are away, patients' calls and visits should be covered. Find out who provides that coverage—a colleague in the same office or system is probably preferable to someone in a random emergency room.

You need to have an interview and a hands-on exam from time to time, especially if you are not feeling well or find a lump or a spot. You should have a few screening tests, too, to find cracks in your engine block before something breaks down. The purpose is to find what's wrong so that you can *do* something about it. Although screening takes a little time, early diagnosis and treatment can save your capabilities and even your life.

Here are six screening tests for men and seven for women that are aimed at keeping you from unnecessary suffering. I am reminded of the rueful comment by fabled Stanford Law School professor, John Kaplan, who said, "I was asked to make a list of all the faculty members broken down by age and sex. Everyone was on it."

Keep in mind that there are inherent harms and benefits to any screening test, especially ones with results that are difficult to interpret, such as the Prostate Specific Antigen (PSA). You and your doctor should decide together whether to start or continue screenings.

I would like to highlight three of the tests:

If your **blood pressure** is edging up, you should have it taken more often than yearly.

If your **blood sugar** is up even a little bit, weight loss and exercise can help prevent damage to your heart, brain, eyes, and kidneys—anywhere you have arteries (and that is everywhere). People of color are at higher risk from high blood sugar.

Since about half of women and a quarter of men over fifty will break a bone because of osteoporosis, it is important to get a **bone mineral density test** every one to three years and to eat a diet rich in calcium and vitamin D (sunshine increases vitamin D only a little).

IMPORTANT SCREENING TESTS FOR ADULTS *(Always check with your doctor first.)*		
Test For	For Whom	How Often If You Feel Well and Are Well
Blood pressure	All adults	Every 1–2 years
Cholesterol	All adults	Every 5 years
Blood sugar	All adults over 50	Every 2–3 years
Breast cancer (mammogram)	All women over 50	Mammogram if over 50 or *earlier* if in special risk groups. Every year; check with your doctor about self-exam instructions

IMPORTANT SCREENING TESTS FOR ADULTS *(Always check with your doctor first.)*		
Cervical cancer	All women	Under 30, every year; over 30, check with your doctor
Prostate cancer	All men over 55	Decide with your doctor
Gastrointestinal bleeding	All adults over 50	Stool test for blood every year; direct exam every 5 years, or sooner if stool test is positive
Osteoporosis (bone mineral density scan)	Women over 60; men over 65	Every 2–5 years
Glaucoma	All adults over 40	Every 3–5 years (more often if very nearsighted or African American)

A medical tune-up should also include thoughtful attention and conversation, advice (about exercise, smoking, safer sex, and the like), instructions, perhaps medications, and a review of your immunizations.

Immunizations tend to be under-appreciated and over-feared, yet they are major health-, cost-, and life-savers. Look at influenza immunizations. Influenza is nothing to sneeze at, partly because it doesn't really involve sneezes. The disease often lays people low for one to three weeks, off work. It makes you stuffy, feverish, and achy. You cough day and all night, are weak, sometimes have nausea and vomiting, may be short of breath, and may develop pneumonia.

You are likely to distribute the misery to family, friends, and perfect strangers. Influenza is more likely to kill younger people, including children, than older ones. You should get flu shots each year because the viruses change every year. Although, like all vaccines, the shots don't provide perfect protection, when the vaccine and circulating virus match well, flu can be reduced in your community by 70 to 90 percent. (If mismatched vaccines and viruses occur, protection may only be 50 percent, but some protection is better than none.) Importantly and despite myths, *flu shots do not give you the flu.* The virus in the shot is dead. It doesn't even contain whole virus particles. Material from the shot cannot replicate nor spread. You can get a fever and sore arm as your body ramps up to fight the disease, but that is *not* the flu. Period.

Getting a "shingles" shot should also be on your docket if you are over sixty. If you have dear ones in that age bracket, pass this word to them. Why? Because the risk of getting shingles increases with age, although I know people in their early forties who have had a bout. At least one million people per year in the U.S. get this miserable, blistering, burning rash that can destroy vision. A shingles shot decreases by half your chance of getting shingles from the chicken pox virus (Herpes zoster) that got stored along your spinal cord when you had "the chicks," as our daughter Sarah called it when she was little. Even if the shot doesn't protect you completely and you do get shingles, your skin involvement will be far less severe, and the risk of shingles-related pain and disability will be lessened by about two thirds. That pain and disability could otherwise go on for months or years. The United States Centers for Disease Control and other immunization specialists agree that you should get the shingles shot *even if you have had the shingles.* The idea is to boost your immunity because your body obviously doesn't have quite enough resistance on its own.

You only need to get the shingles shot once in your lifetime.

You need the third of my three favorite immunizations, Tdap (Tetanus, diphtheria, and pertussis), once after childhood in order to keep your immunity up to snuff. Avid gardeners take note: tetanus bacteria spores can live in the soil for forty years, so any deep wound could be infected. In the United States, tetanus (or lockjaw, well named because jaw spasms herald the disease and may last for months) is fatal for about one out of five infected people. It is a terrible death, in convulsions, by suffocating, or from heart disease. Antibiotics don't touch the bacteria, which secrete toxins that injure tissues. Pertussis—whooping cough (well named because of the sound of its desperate coughing gasps) or the "ninety-day cough"—is having an uncomfortable resurgence in adults as their immunity from childhood shots wanes. Pertussis doesn't kill many people, but it is exhausting to suffer through. Diphtheria organisms stimulate the formation of a membrane in your throat that is hard to clear. Five to ten percent of people who get diphtheria die of it, partly because your heart can be affected, too. One shot—a booster Tdap—can prevent all of these risks and ordeals for you and those close to you.

IMPORTANT IMMUNIZATIONS *(Always check with your doctor.)*		
Decreases Risk Of	Who and When	How Often
Influenza	All adults	Every year
Shingles	All adults over 60, unless a live weakened virus would be a problem	Once
Tetanus, diphtheria, pertussis	All adults	Once after childhood

Now that you are caught up on tests and shots, it is time to get more specific about your very own particular body. Fill in these blanks—or as many as you can. Don't make up the answers. Drop by the drugstore to get your blood pressure, cholesterol, and blood glucose (sugar) checked if you don't have a medical home or you haven't been keeping track. Get out the tape measure, too.

34

MY BODY
Blood pressure_____(normal is 120/80mmHg or below; pre-hypertension is 120-139/80; hypertension is 140/90 or above. We now know that the numbers above the line and below the line are significant. Hypertension—high blood pressure— doesn't mean that you feel "hyper" or "tense," but it causes your arteries to narrow and can rob your brain with a stroke, cripple your kidneys, or lead to a heart attack if it goes untreated.)
Waist circumference at your belly button_____(above 88 cm or 35 inches for women, and above 102 cm or 40 inches for men, is likely to be too high. If this is you, join the majority: 2/3 of adults in the United States are overweight. Bear in mind that the higher the number, the higher your risk of diabetes, hypertension, and heart and brain attacks.)
Cholesterol
Total_____(should be under 200 mg/dl) High Density Lipoprotein (HDL)_____(should be over 50 mg/dl) Low Density Lipoprotein (LDL)_____(should be under 100 mg/dl) Blood glucose (sugar)_____(normal is 70-100 mg/dl)
Women
Date of last mammogram_____(screening should be yearly if you are over 50; ask your doctor about screening if you are between 40 and 49) Date of last cervical cancer check_____(every year until you turn 30, then less often if tests are negative)

Men
Have you discussed getting a PSA or a digital rectal exam with your physician and followed up on the advice? ❑ Yes ❑ No

Men and women
Do you know how often to schedule a colonoscopy, and is it scheduled? ❑ Yes ❑ No If not, explain why not ("being chicken" isn't a good answer):
Are your immunizations up to date, including influenza; Tetanus, diphtheria, pertussis (Tdap); and shingles (if indicated)? ❑ Yes ❑ No
Are you eating or drinking 1,000 to 1,200 mg of calcium per day? (Milk has about 300 mg per cup, somewhat less than collards, more than spinach, and almost twice the amount of 3 oz of calcium-set tofu) ❑ Yes ❑ No
Are you getting about 1,000 International Units (IU) of vitamin D per day? (Milk has 100 IU per cup.) ❑ Yes ❑ No
For anyone who has broken a bone after age 50, anyone who is older than 65, and anyone who is very slender or has a family history of bone disease: Have you talked with your clinician and will have (or already had) a bone mineral density scan? ❑ Yes ❑ No
For anyone over 40: have you had a glaucoma test in the last three to five years? ❑ Yes ❑ No
Do you get at least a half hour of exercise at least five days a week that increases your heart rate over 110? (All things being equal, at least some of the exercise should put a load on your bones and stretch your tendons.) ❑ Yes ❑ No

You can refresh your healthy body awareness by reviewing this chart and by filling in new answers. Taking care of your priceless body is a big part of your fatigue treatment and prevention.

THE STATE OF YOUR SPIRIT

Physicist-philosopher Albert Einstein opined, "Not everything that counts can be counted, and not everything that can be counted counts." You have just taken care of several items—how you are feeling and doing and how your body measures up—that count *and* can be counted.

In addition to your physical health, your spirits count—a lot—and they may be harder to gauge. Spirits are changeable and can be puzzling. Mine certainly are! Sometimes when a driver grabs the parking place I had been stalking, I sweetly think, "Ah, must be in a hurry or having a bad day, poor thing." Other times I'd just as soon ram 'im.

The term "spirit" is fascinating in itself. When physicians refer to the act of breathing, we describe inspiration and expiration, or breathing in and breathing out. These movements supply life-giving oxygen and remove carbon dioxide, a waste product of metabolism. In Hebrew, *ruach* means both breath and spirit. "Inspiration" can allude to inventions and ideas as the spirit enlivens you and leads to something new. "Expired," of course, means dead—no spirit left.

The next part of your checkup is about your spirits. I'm sure that even this huge list may not be long enough to capture your many-sided, fluid spirit, but give it a whirl, and check off the descriptions that fit you. This "ballot" comes from all the listening I've done over the years. The idea is to begin to understand the way you feel—body and soul—so you will be able to apply the Fatigue Prescription to yourself as you really are.

Lean back and stretch tall. Be open and willing for the "aha" of awareness. After you check the boxes and add to the list, if you wish, you might want to go for a walk and chew over your answers, along with a companion or an apple. It's a good idea to distill the list into three to five descriptions that capture your spirit. High, low, sturdy, wavering, or any combination.

MY SPIRIT	
Low	Anxious
Great	Good
Awakening	Buoyant
Neutral	Barely OK
Optimistic	Fair
Disillusioned	Positive
Happy	Mixed
Starved	Too serious
Uneasy	Hopeful
Stifled	Connected
Trying hard	Beat up
Stretched thin	Doing fine but I want some help
Way too tired	Coping but frustrated
Excited	Hurtin'
Panic stricken	Days and days of no fun
Career tumult	Grateful
Fearful	About the happiest I've ever been

MY SPIRIT	
Like a bag of carrots at the grocery	In transition
I *wish* I felt as good as a bag of carrots; I feel like a mushed rutabaga	Looking forward to something special
Flexible	It'll be tough to go back after maternity leave/vacation
Overflowing with energy	Happy with my choices
Ambivalent	Recovering
Under-appreciated	How bad could it be? I'm going on vacation!
It depends	Other
MY SPIRIT: A SUMMARY	

YOUR RELATIONSHIPS

Relationships are major factors in your health and renewal because they can be sources of peace and support—or war and destruction. They are therefore a high priority, and I'll mention them several times throughout this book. In this section, after I describe some difficult relationships, I will show why *all* relationships are so significant.

A couple of years ago, a physician's wife told a RENEW workshop, "I'm married to an internist. I'm basically a single mom." Another wife said, "My husband and I have four children. He is busy at the office day and night. He has had no influence on our kids." A man who heard that remarked, "Oh yes, your husband definitely has influence on his kids—by his absence."

Some relationships can suck you dry; others can agitate you so much that your energy evaporates into steam. Unreasonable, perpetual demanders can irritate and flatten you at the same time, because there is no pleasing them. There is also a category of "help-rejecting complainers." No matter what you do or arrange for them, it just doesn't work out well. Jamie once went to monumental efforts to get special dental care for a patient who had no money. After a series of appointments didn't work out, she missed the last appointment "because my girdle wasn't clean enough." For a dental office? Jamie threw in the towel.

With so many examples of bad relationships, why do we bother getting into them at all? What's the big deal about bonding?

It seems likely that people were made to band together. It would have been tough, way back when, to face a saber-toothed tiger alone. It would have been hard to keep the home fire burning alone. It has always taken two to tango or to procreate. From the standpoint of survival, people who work (and play) well together are the ones who weather the elements, eat enough, and help societies flourish.

Relationships are universal. Groups of bushmen in the Kalahari Desert sustain their links to each other with stories, visits, and gifts because they desperately need each other during disasters. You aren't so different. You have electronic and in-person social networks that provide career, health, friendship, planning, and information networks. By now, you may have come to realize that technology can separate and isolate as much as it may bring people together, however. Playing games on the Internet is not the same as seeing each other eye to eye, having a chat, or sharing a snack in person. Busy schedules may put you in contact with many people, but that doesn't mean you'll build relationships that are strong enough to depend on when adversity hammers.

Think of all of your energy-giving connections. Remember teachers and friends who have encouraged you (I will cover Encouragers in greater detail in a later chapter). Back to Latin: e*n* = in, *cor* = heart. When people *encourage* you, they put their heart into yours. Other connections give energy, too. My husband Jamie made a list for himself of "patients who make me smile." He realized that he wasn't as tired at the end of a day when any of them had an appointment. A financial advisor told me that what she misses most about losing her job at the bank is her pals. She yearns for the coffee and water cooler stories, dumb jokes, and cheerleading that renewed her vitality. To fill in some of those relationship gaps, she has increased her volunteering with neighborhood school kids.

To help keep an eye on the health of your assorted connections, Psychiatrist Michael Myers suggests being aware of some danger signals. See if you are aware of any of these as you apply them to your family, friends, colleagues, clients, and others you have relationships with:

- Tensions
- Withdrawing
- Stilted or superficial conversations (you soft-pedal around or avoid more important subjects, such as money or sex)
- Denying over-commitment to work (including volunteering) or other outside-your-home activities.
- Wrestling for control
- Depression

You signaled some of your own relationship issues in the Renew-O-Meter. But now it's time to get more in-depth. Unwind and make yourself at home, wherever you are. Let's see how you're doing with others and the status of your energy-giving bonds. Your answers to the questions can help you set your goals and chart your course.

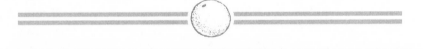

MY RELATIONSHIPS
Be specific about important connections (parents, siblings, partner, children, friends, colleagues, clients, and yourself), and check the appropriate boxes.
My important relationships are basically pleasant. ❏ Yes ❏ No
My important relationships are basically pleasant, but there are some chronic sore spots. ❏ Yes ❏ No If so, list some

MY RELATIONSHIPS
I feel as if I might be dropping some important balls. ❑ Yes ❑ No If so, which ones? (Marriage, customers, pals?)
I never have enough hours in the day to enjoy all my close relationships. ❑ Yes ❑ No Comment:
Do I withdraw from others, or do they withdraw from me? Circle the answer.
My relationships could be much better. ❑ Yes ❑ No If so, in what way?
How do you feel about yourself these days (yourself being your most important relationship)? Check one: ❑ Yuck ❑ Not great ❑ Neutral (pluses = minuses) ❑ Okay, generally ❑ Mainly positive ❑ Great! I love myself ❑ Other

YOUR LEARNING CHECKUP

Learning is an essential part of vanquishing fatigue. Look at what you have already learned and how far you have come!

Learning works against fatigue partly because it saves wear and tear. You learn where to get the electronic parking meter cards so you don't have to schlep a ton of quarters. Night courses in psychology and communication may help save your sanity or composure during your children's adolescence or your parents' decline.

Learning has advantages beyond its practical value, too. It can bring on a peak experience, the *YES!* of mastering a geometry proof, a stick shift, angel food cake, or a ten-foot putt. It can help you get what you want, as in learning about interviewing when you go for a job interview and negotiating when you go for a raise.

You may learn how friendship works, as I did during my times of trouble. Paola Gianturco is a college classmate who broke every mold in her business and publishing careers. She called me time and again to check on how I was getting along as blow after blow fell during the year and a half when I lost so much—my parents, my husband's health, jobs, and a safe home. Finally I said, "I am no fun. I am not Sparkle Plenty any more. I can barely get through the day. Why do you keep calling me?" She said, "I am your friend." "Oh," I said. Until then, I had thought friends were for fun, entertainment, parties, and games.

Learning can also be an antidote to suffering. As Merlin puts it in *The Once and Future King*:

> The best thing for being sad...is to learn something....
> You may grow old and trembling in your anatomies...
> you may miss your only love, you may see the world
> about you devastated by evil lunatics or know your
> honor trampled in the sewers of baser minds. There's

only one thing for it then: to learn. Learn why the world
wags and what wags it....Learning is the thing for you.

Most learning happens outside of school. You say "live and
learn" with a sigh when you forget your umbrella anytime in April.
You learn when you travel. Who knew that every rock and tree in
Bhutan has a spirit? You can learn while getting some exercise and
making some Vitamin D, like a bird aficionado I know who hikes,
spots owls, and listens to university lectures on CDs.

However gained, learning is refreshing. It provides everyday
handiness and perspective. It is a welcome tonic that can help you
evaluate and perhaps re-tool your treadmill.

Of course, learning can be difficult, especially if you think you
know it all. Pioneer scientist Claude Bernard wrote, "It is what
we think we know already that often prevents us from learning."
Fifteenth-century experts thought they knew that Filippo
Brunelleschi could never build the massive yet graceful Duomo that
defines Florence's skyline because he would have to deforest Italy
to get enough wood for the scaffolding. He went ahead anyway
and built it without scaffolding. For generations, scientists and the
public thought they knew that peptic ulcers were caused by stress
or excess acid until Australians Marshall and Warren proved in the
1980's that a bacterium is to blame in most cases. You hear almost
every week about an innocent lookalike who was jailed because a
jury "knew" she was the culprit, but DNA fingers the real perpe-
trator. "Knowing" isn't the same as "learning."

Just as authorities throughout time have needed to unlearn
cherished beliefs, you may need to reprogram hard-won or wrong
lessons. A prison chaplain recalled that as a little boy he was never
allowed to cry. If he "tuned up," as his father called it, his father
beat him until the big muscular man got tired. Years later, the

chaplain found that he needed to burrow into and air his feelings in order to do his job well. He had to set aside a lifetime of suppressing his emotions to do so.

Since learning is a lifelong quest, ask yourself:

MY LEARNING
What have I learned in the last two weeks or so that astounded me?
When I read the paper or a blog or catch the news, what subjects intrigue me (not including sports, advice columns, and the comics)?
Do I need to **un**learn anything? Perhaps about my relationships? Or my scheduling? Or any assumptions?

YOUR ATTITUDE CHECKUP

Everyone has attitudes. They live in you and tend to persist unchecked unless you take charge. They can shape your appearance—recall the sullen smirk of someone you caught in the act. Grounded in emotion, attitudes show up in your body language, words, and behavior. Attitudes are your outlooks at the same time that they mirror you.

Attitudes, along with values, are the most important choices you can make. It may not be as easy as "snapping out of it," but you *can* choose your attitudes. As Viktor Frankl, a psychiatrist and Holocaust death camp survivor, said, "Everything can be taken from a man but one thing: the last of the human freedoms—to choose one's attitude."

In a classic study of attitude and grit, psychotherapist Lillian Rubin in *The Transcendent Child* recorded the stories of eight remarkable people who crafted reasonably pleasant adult lives despite having childhoods marked by brutal abuse, poverty, and mental illness. From childhood on, unlike their siblings, who fell down and stayed down, Rubin's subjects fell down seven times and got up eight. Rubin reported that they shared several features: They chose to separate themselves from the maelstrom around them by living at the periphery of their families. They developed outside interests and attracted helping hands. They were fiercely independent and tenacious. They constructed their own versions of their own stories that put them in a U-turn mode, away from their families' downhill slides. Above all, they chose their attitude: not to be victims.

Attitudes are like colors. There is a full spectrum. Being optimistic or pessimistic, open or closed, feeling can-do or can't-do are the extremes, but there are countless shades in between. Attitudes can vary with circumstance, such as your energy level and how tired you are. At the end of some days, I look at a pile of work and slump with a "NO WAY" attitude. The next morning, after a good night's sleep, I charge through the pile like a house afire. By now I know not to bother worrying about the pile, because my attitude will shift in the morning when it *is* a better day.

According to current research, it looks as if attitudes may also make a difference in health. This is no wonder when you consider the ways your body and mind influence each other. Research over the past quarter century has shown some of the burdens of pessimism. A 2002 study by Maruta et al. showed that those who are convinced "it's going to last forever" and "it's going to undermine everything" have "poorer physical health, are prone to depression, [and] have a less adequately functioning immune system...than others." This study showed that people who held a pessimistic outlook for thirty years (from about age thirty to sixty) had "poorer physical and mental function compared to optimists or people with mixed pessimism and optimism." They had more physical and mental limitations, less vitality, and more limited work and social functioning than the others. The optimists in the study had a 50 percent decreased risk of early death. These results might be partly explained by the brain's effect on the immune system, plus patients' depression and learned helplessness. Attitudes about health care itself may be an additional part of the story, since pessimists generally expect less of health care and also seek it less. In any event, the point is that feeling bad can be a self-fulfilling prophesy.

Other studies have also shown that optimism is associated with longer life. "Association" is not the same as "causation," of course. There's no guarantee of a long life for optimists, since heredity, good sense, education, economic status, and luck play a role. But take a look at two studies. The *UC Berkeley Wellness Letter* reported that in one small town, long-term research focused on people of comparable race, gender, health, morale, and loneliness.

Those "over fifty who viewed aging as a positive experience lived an average of 7.5 years longer than those who did not." Looking at deaths from heart attacks and strokes, another study by Giltay, et al. followed almost one thousand men and women from ages sixty-five to eighty-five for about nine years. After adjusting for age, gender, illnesses, and smoking, the investigators found that people who were high on the optimism scale had about one-fourth the risk of death from cardiovascular causes and about one-half the risk of death from any cause during the study period as the pessimists. Perhaps optimists live a self-fulfilling prophecy, too: they expect to live long and therefore take better care of themselves.

As you've probably guessed, I am an optimist—which, I've been told, can be irritating. But being a tough-minded optimist has gotten me through some pretty hard times, and I've found that pessimism can be paralyzing. As Yale professor of molecular biophysics and biochemistry, Harold J. Morowitz, said in the journal, *Hospital Practice:*

> Well, you grumps and grouches and dyspeptics out there—your cover has been blown. There is nothing so intellectually deep about your pessimism. Indeed, it could be regarded as a rationalization or easy way out. Your very gloom about the future may be providing you with a reason for not putting forth all the work necessary to overcome the decay that you envision. Recall the words of Henry David Thoreau: "Men will lie on their backs talking about the fall of man and never make an effort to get up."

Look at how well you're doing already! You are choosing to get up so you can regain your sense of purpose and fulfillment.

This is the last part of your own checkup. It is about your attitude toward *yourself.*

When our church was redesigning its building and programs, our minister Pam Shortridge sent the congregation a letter suggesting that we take stock of ourselves before launching into the overhaul, to make sure we were up to taking the risks and following through with substantial changes. We didn't all ace the test, but we found—quite to our surprise—that we had good-sized reservoirs of oomph, no matter how tired or worried we felt right then. We thought we could do it—and we did it.

Here is the questionnaire Pam distributed. You may just want to take a look at it and think about it, or you may want to try "yes/no/maybe." You may even score each item from 0–10 (low to high). The idea is to take a close look at yourself and see, as you shape your attitudes, where you most need the Fatigue Prescription.

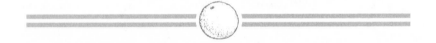

MY ATTITUDE
I can handle discomfort. ❑ Yes ❑ No ❑ Maybe
I can handle not knowing how things will turn out. ❑ Yes ❑ No ❑ Maybe
I trust that something new and more appropriate will emerge from the chaos. ❑ Yes ❑ No ❑ Maybe
I am open to new ways of being and doing things. ❑ Yes ❑ No ❑ Maybe
I can envision something new and help make it a reality. ❑ Yes ❑ No ❑ Maybe
I can continue to grow and learn. ❑ Yes ❑ No ❑ Maybe

Rumi, the thirteenth-century Sufi poet, jurist, and theologian, wrote about what you face as you gear up to renew.

GUEST HOUSE

This being human is a guest house
Every morning a new arrival.
A joy, a depression, a meanness,
some momentary awareness comes
as an unexpected visitor.
Welcome and entertain them all!
Even if they are a crowd of sorrows,
who violently sweep your house
empty of its furniture,
still treat each guest honorably.
He may be clearing you out for some new delight.
The dark thought, the sham, the malice,
meet them at the door laughing,
and invite them in.
Be grateful for whoever comes,
because each has been sent
as a guide from beyond.

(Translated by Coleman Barks)

The next chapter gives some reasons to be grateful for these guides.

CHAPTER 3

THE PROBLEMS
AND THE PROMISE

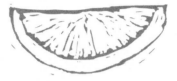

"I am all for progress. It is just change that I don't like."
—Mark Twain

Now that you have had some *aha*s, you may feel ready to start making some shifts. But wait! You're way over the hump in the Fatigue Prescription diagnostic work-up, yet there is a bit more to do. Only four more quick questions remain. One deals with what you would like to get from the Fatigue Prescription. I ask that because RENEW and this book are based in part on adult learning theory. It infers that you are independent, experienced, self-motivated, and oriented toward solving everyday problems. This question puts adult learning theory into practice. The remaining three questions are about change, since change is afoot as your awareness and reflections blossom after your winter—or longer—of fatigue.

But what if change isn't your cup of latte? That's a problem, because sensible change brings promise. I'm not talking about taking a flamethrower to your life, but rather helping those flickering embers of purpose and joy catch fire.

If you don't relish change, you're not alone. The majority of people sense the need to make transitions but are adept at resisting actually making them.

At a convention of entrepreneurs, close to 100 percent voted a vigorous "yes" when asked if they love or like change or enjoy making change happen. In other groups, the "yes" votes plummet. Maybe 10–15 percent of people acknowledge their willingness to receive change when it comes along. They like the stimulation but don't want to be in the forefront. Another 20–40 percent tolerate change, asking copious questions along the way. The remaining people shrink or wail at the thought of change and may fight it tooth and nail.

The last two groups include almost everyone. But change will come. A contemporary Korean poet observed:

> Flowers bloom. They are not the same as last year's.
> Flowers fall, not in the same spot as last year's.
> *Nothing in the world stays the same.*

Why does change seem so daunting? For one thing, it doesn't necessarily come in manageable sizes. Like the bowls of porridge in *Goldilocks*, change may be medium, large, or small. Baby Bear change can mean tinkering—like trying a new version of a recipe or a new route to work. Mama Bear change may take some stretching, even discomfort, and often involves other people and politics—designing a new curriculum or fixing a system to solve customer service complaints, for example. Papa Bear change is often downright unsettling and involves everyone who cares about it—consider job loss, divorce, bad sickness, or death. Major change is particularly hard because it often requires coping with unknowns and ambiguity. Even good Papa Bear change can cause strain—marriage, a new school, a new job. Sometimes the whole bowl of porridge gets dumped right on top of your head, raisins and all.

Also, change does not necessarily come in small doses. My life collapsed in eighteen months with a whole series of heartbreaking losses. In an even more sudden one-two-three punch, the day after a friend of ours was told he had cancer, he was asked to officiate at a friend's funeral, and two days later another destabilizing force occurred when a foreign student houseguest started a week's stay.

Where do you sit right now with possible changes (work, friends, neighborhood, duties, goals, yourself)? Try these questions:

IS CHANGE ON MY HORIZON? *Check appropriate boxes:*	
Way too much on my plate	
Need to change	
Want to change	
Don't want to change	
I'm ambivalent about change	
Must change	
Should I change?	
Can I change?	
Change is tough; how do I do it?	

If you are feeling a tug or a push toward making a change, your contrarian tendencies may ask, "Why bother?"

BENEFITS OF THE FATIGUE PRESCRIPTION

It may seem counterintuitive, but resisting change brings fatigue. You are a capable person with good things happening in your life and plenty to look forward to—but fatigue melts your interests and commitments into slush. You make mistakes because you hurry to get *some*thing done. Your modus operandi robs you of the satisfaction and joy you should feel. It is no surprise that you are tired.

But as you begin to unload your fatigue, you will be able to change your attitude about change. The goal is to proceed beyond merely *enduring* change and to begin to seek or welcome change and consider it a natural, even exhilarating part of life.

The idea is to stay upright and flexible while you develop goals and deadlines. A flight attendant once told me, "I've given myself until the end of the year to get a transfer to Los Angeles instead of San Francisco. If I don't get it, I'm going to move to L.A. anyway and just get a new job. That'd be a lot of change all at once, but I don't mind. The scarier it is, the more fun it is, like downhill skiing!"

When you're suffering from fatigue, you feel like a dry sponge. You take up space, but all the juice has been squeezed out of you.

Fatigue isn't only bad for your feelings; it is bad for your health. You may have aches and pains, upset stomach, a racing heart, rising blood pressure, ballooning weight, sleeplessness or an inability to get out of bed, and the urge to start smoking again—all related to fatigue. I've seen headaches, backaches, rashes, and flares of chronic illnesses such as asthma and diabetes that are directly attributable to fatigue. Fatigue can also lead to inattentiveness, slow reaction times, and impaired judgment.

Does any of this sound familiar?

I do not make promises lightly, and yet I promise that you can heal. One simple first step is to give yourself a break and remove voluntary toxins: stop drinking alcohol in excess and quit smoking.

Stopping alcohol abuse before scars set in allows your liver to regain its abilities to cleanse your blood, make and store important vitamins, manufacture proteins that are essential to life, and store nutrients. Decreasing alcohol intake helps your brain, too, so your thinking sharpens and your relationships and work improve. Lung function can return to normal if you stop smoking before fibrous tissue predominates. Cancer and heart disease risks drop when you quit smoking, too.

I am saying stop digging holes. This applies not only to noxious agents, but to food as well. For one thing, you have to watch your timing. Dark chocolate may be good for your heart and lift your spirits, but if you eat chunks just before bedtime, its stimulants can shrink your forty winks to twenty. In addition, its chemicals can trigger migraines or heartburn.

Another thing to be aware of is portion control. "Portion control" doesn't mean you have to stop eating. It means to eat a little of everything and a lot of nothing. The fact that peanut butter may contain aflatoxins (made by the mold that can grow on peanut shells) does not negate its high-protein nutritional value. But afla-toxins are powerful carcinogens. That doesn't mean you should stop eating peanut butter; it means you shouldn't eat it morning, noon, and night (or if looks moldy). Sodium is another example. Cutting back on salt can lower your blood pressure and slenderize your puffy ankles as the excess fluid that sodium attracts floats out in your urine, courtesy of your kidneys.

REAPING BENEFITS REQUIRES RISKS

Managing your fatigue means that you will need to take some risks. This, too, can be a challenge. Not everyone likes to take risks.

Why bother taking risks? It is not just to "get out of the comfort zone," as Bill Walsh, famed football coach, said. That advice may be hard to swallow, since it takes a good deal of hard work to get *into* a comfort zone. The zone isn't forever, however. Comfort can become tiresome. You may ignore your goals and values in order to stay comfortable. Or a competitor may poke holes in your pillow of repose and let your stuffing out.

According to University of Southern California psychologist Leo F. Buscaglia, "The person who risks nothing, does nothing, has nothing, is nothing, and becomes nothing...He simply cannot learn and feel and change and grow and love and live...He's forfeited his freedom. Only the person who risks is truly free."

Part of venturing out of your comfort zone is to augment your awareness, just as you are doing right now. Sometimes awareness is almost musical. At a RENEWing conversation a few years ago, we were discussing how people knew that they were tired and might need to push out of their comfort zones. One young man said that he sighed more often than usual. When he mentioned sighing, a chorus of sighs rippled around the group. It was such a poignant moment that we sat silently for a few moments and let the sighs sink in. Over the next few weeks we kept track of when, where, and why we sighed. This helped pinpoint our sources of fatigue. In epidemiological terms, our "index case" (the first one who came to our attention) realized that he was on overload. He spoke with colleagues about ways to manage his work better. He also changed his route home so he could enjoy the sunsets on a winding road instead of barreling along a freeway. The trip took a bit longer but his sighs subsided.

You may feel desperate at the thought of taking a risk. But keep in mind that taking a chance isn't necessarily a sudden event. William Bridges, a former English professor and careful observer, suggests that the process of making transitions has sequential elements. External change leads to internal transitions in three phases: an *ending* and an acknowledgement of that ending, a *neutral zone* that allows reflection and serendipity to blossom into surprising developments, and a *beginning* of life's next chapter. This is one reason why taking a chance may take months or years of preparation.

Depending on the speed of your evolution, by the time you make your move, the limb you climb out on might not seem so long or wobbly. You may even enjoy the view!

Even if it may not seem like it, you do have the gumption to crawl out on that limb and adjust some of your customary ways. Before I discuss how to do that, take a minute to reflect on what makes you feel like you aren't up to the task. Here are some thoughts on change I've collected over the years:

MY ATTITUDES ABOUT CHANGE
I'm too depressed. I can only see opportunities through "blue" colored glasses.
It's too hard to change.
I don't like to feel vulnerable.
I'm a slave to having power or I'm a slave to money.
I'm hooked on doing public service. I can't imagine anything besides being a caregiver.
Others don't want me to change.
I've seen others attempt change and fail.
I don't have enough willpower to sustain change.

MY ATTITUDES ABOUT CHANGE
It's easier to complain.
I'm stubborn.
I'm too old.
I'm afraid.

Do any of these sound familiar? Add to this list your own reasons for not changing:

MY FAVORITE REASONS FOR NOT CHANGING

GOING BEYOND BALANCE

Now for the shocker: if your goal is to overcome fatigue, *balance is not your ticket.*

WHAT?

I know what you're thinking: everyone, I mean *every*one, talks about balance! Don't get me wrong; there is nothing *bad* about balance. Entire divisions, departments, and companies are devoted to it. Nonetheless, going for balance has two huge disadvantages. One: achieving balance is way too hard. Two: balance just isn't enough to sustain you over the long haul. It is *necessary* but not *sufficient*. How come?

Of course people rely on physical balance at all times, from walking down the street to changing a ceiling light bulb to mountain climbing. From a human developmental and repair perspective, just see how hard it is to attain balance. It takes babies a year or more to take their triumphant first step. Think, too, of a stranger, friend, or parent with a brain injury such as a stroke try to recover. Helping hands, grab bars, walkers, and canes may be called in to provide support before their triumphal first step toward improved balance.

Even when you are good at a feat, however, losing your balance, especially at high speed, is a shock to your system. It is discombobulating and can cause severe trauma. And emotional balance works the same way, which is why you need more than balance to keep on getting healthy and staying healthy. You need anchors that endure because balance is a moment-to-moment matter.

Satisfying as it is, balance is temporary. A university department chair pointed out that balance falsely implies an "optimum," that is, a *best* way. The trouble is, the definition of "best" is always changing, whether in sports or the stock market.

Let's get beyond balance. You want your days to have some zip and zing. You want to be sturdy, creative, and productive. You want to feel good. You can achieve all that by puting the Prescription into practice.

WHAT WE NEED IS HERE

Geese appear high over us,
pass, and the sky closes. Abandon,
as in love or sleep, holds
them to their way, clear
in the ancient faith: what we need
is here. And we pray, not
for new earth or heaven, but to be
quiet in heart, and in eye,
clear. What we need is here.

—Wendell Berry

PART TWO

THE RENEWING REMEDY

CHAPTER 4

THE FOUR STEPS

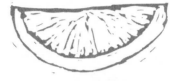

You've got to have a dream. If you don't have a dream,
how you gonna have a dream come true?

—*South Pacific*

There are many ways to fill the Fatigue Prescription. You can
do it by yourself or with others. You can do it in silence or with
soft, surround-sound music. Sometimes you fill the Prescription
out loud; other times you do it on paper. Hearing others' stories
reminds you that you are not the only one who is tired—and if
others can revise, you can, too. An experienced RENEWer said,
"Through listening, you discover more common ground than you
would ever have imagined."

Before you begin the renewing process, make some arrangements that will help you use the tools in this book efficiently:

Find a pleasant, calm, safe place where you will be comfortable
settling down, on and off, over several days.

Set up your surroundings so you'll be able to concentrate.

Make sure your mind is wide open to new ideas. Some of the dust will need to get swept away, and some thoughts set in concrete will need to be remodeled.

Make sure your mind is sticky, too, so new notions can land and become the foundation for new structures.

Now you're ready to get started. It is time to become—and remain—the person you want to be.

STEP ONE: AWARENESS

Awareness comes first in the Prescription because you have to know what is going on around and within yourself before you can do anything about it. Awareness often starts with prickles and inklings—or sometimes a sledgehammer—that beg for your attention. Once you up periscope, you may realize that your fatigue isn't all your own doing. I heard two nurses talking recently. The first said, "I just want to collapse from this fatigue. I have millions of lists. I'm constantly triaging my whole life, not just at work." The second replied, "Your fatigue isn't the whole picture. Sometimes you're in a situation with a hospital changing hands, or cutbacks, or an administration that doesn't 'get it', and it's out of your control. It isn't *your* fatigue; it's someone else's added on to yours."

In addition to being aware of external factors, pay attention to yourself—your sighs and groans, or the silence when your whistling or humming stops. What other signs of trouble do you regularly display? Are they related to certain people or situations?

In Chapter 2 you listed your signs of trouble. Now settle back and let's think about what brings them on.

SIGN OF TROUBLE	
Who Does It to Me?	
What Does It to Me?	
When Does It Tend to Happen?	

The patterns of your signs of trouble can also give you clues about the negative effects of your fatigue. In addition to recognizing who might be imposing their fatigue on you, it's wise to start thinking about who is feeling the effects of *your* fatigue. Who is at the bottom of your downspout: your spouse, partner, colleagues, children, the woman behind the counter at the dry cleaner?

Relationships may falter not only because of toxic interactions, but also because of absenteeism. A celebrated innovator and president of a think tank told me about the night he returned from a continent-spanning string of speeches. His teenage daughter set the dinner table for three—herself, her brother, and her mother. She hadn't even noticed that her dad was home! He got the picture, and he decided that very day to step down from the presidency. He wanted to be present for his family, not just for his office and fame, and he saw how at odds his lifestyle was with his real purpose. Like him, awareness may come to you with all the subtlety of a thunderbolt.

Sometimes awareness means examining comfortable patterns to see if they are serving you well. Often, for example, what you assume is a groove (a good thing) is actually a rut (a not-so-good thing) that is lulling you into complacency.

A few years back, California Pacific Medical Center's Values Action Committee described grooves and ruts. Members decided that being in a groove gives you a distinct sense of flow, like the flow of water over and around a rock. You stride. Things fall into place. It feels good and you feel good about yourself (not complacent but *good*). You look forward to going to work, to climbing the next hill. You have the sense that even little steps are an accomplishment. Joy travels within you when you're in a groove. Life feels like an expedition, a spirited undertaking full of swoops and *wheee*s rather than a plodding journey weighing you down. When you are in a groove, your attitude is up.

A rut makes you slump. You can get three hundred emails a day and have eight meetings on Tuesday from dawn into the night and still be in a rut—a very, very busy rut. You can't see over the edge of the rut; you're afraid even to get close to the edge. Ruts are restricting. A rut may be comfortable, but it's a pinching, diminishing place, an attitude downer.

STEP TWO: REFLECTION

The results of reflection may amaze you. You will be able to understand and integrate more about yourself and why you do the things you do. With reflection, you may decide to forgive yourself for mistakes you have made. This will unlock waves of energy that will refresh your very being. As you think, your purpose will clarify. Reflection will help you refine your purpose, and with it, options and strategies will generate to push you forward.

Setting Yourself Up for Reflection

Reflection methods vary. I suggest you start in the appealing space you created to use with the Prescription. You might engage in formal meditation, shut your eyes and breathe deeply, or gaze at treetops or waves lapping at a shore. If you can't arrange a perfect spot to sit and reflect, fantasize yourself there instead.

Reflection is a new undertaking for many, so lower your expectations and be considerate of yourself. I got comfort from a session on meditation that the Dalai Lama led at Stanford. As he described his technique, he acknowledged that it was hard for him to meditate for much more than twenty minutes. "I start to itch," he reported.

Being practical, you can think when you are on the run, in the car, between meetings, on line at the bank—anywhere! Carry a notebook with a cover design that appeals to you so you'll be more likely to pick it up. Attach a click-top pen to it. Make sure these are small enough to fit in your pocket, purse, or briefcase. If you don't want to use "old fashioned" paper and pen, all kinds of electronic communicators can be great reflection-storage devices as well.

It's easier to think when you set boundaries that give you time to do so. Just because every phone message begs for a speedy return call and every incoming email has two exclamation points doesn't mean you have to reply right then. I have a friend with four children who needed quiet time, so she got a lock for the door to her bathroom, her only refuge. If you have an office door, shut it during your reflection time. Oliver Dutton, a colleague of mine at the American College of Physicians, has an automatic email response message that says: "I check my email every hour on the hour. If you need to contact me before that, here is my phone number." Think about these and other maneuvers that free you from having to be immediately available to everyone at all times.

Subject Matter for Reflection

Without some guideposts, I could obsess or wallow indefinitely in the alcoves of my mind and then wander off into the fog. The following topics provide some markers to follow as you think and dream, and as you pull yourself toward the meaning of your life.

Good Things

When you take some time to think, you will discover that if you try, you can stumble across a fair number of good things that are happening in your life—even little things such as finding a nickel or seeing a rainbow. You can be glad for a compliment or soothing conversation, or you can look back at near misses and bullets dodged. Believe me, *something* is going well for you. Put things into perspective, and then write down some good things. Be specific.

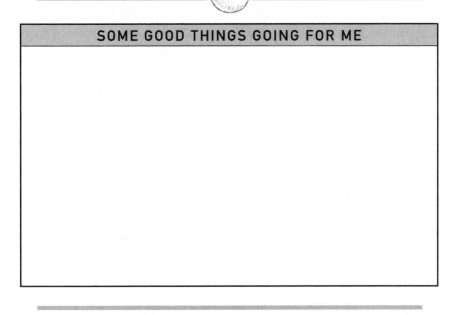

SOME GOOD THINGS GOING FOR ME

Reflecting on good things isn't cheesy or sentimental. It can carry a lot of weight. When a physician friend found himself at a crossroads a few years ago, spinning his wheels and not enjoying much of his life, he spent time thinking about two things: what he loved about medicine and something wonderful that happened every day. He realized that what he loved about medicine was the patients—shutting the examining room door and taking care of people. He re-arranged his practice so that younger partners took on more administrative responsibilities and resigned from a couple of committees. He was also very disciplined about writing down one wonderful thing per day. Some days his standards had to be fairly low, but he always found one wonderful thing. About six months later, he told me, "I am a new man."

People

Some people stick *by* you; others stick *to* you. Who adds to your life? Who detracts? Who energizes you? Who tires you out? One of the best definitions of friendship I know was given to me by a woman who had been a refugee: "A friend is someone who will take you in in the middle of the night when you are running away." Using that description, most of us have rather few friends. Since it takes time to make a friend, tending to them is important. (I'll furnish some time-honored pointers on getting and keeping friends in Chapter 8.)

Priorities

When you reflect on your values, what you consider good and bad and right and wrong, you can start to set priorities. This is crucial, since when everything is a priority, nothing is a priority. Your priorities become not the power sources that give purpose to your life, but rather fuel that you consume, draining your energy bucket until there is not a particle left.

After you spend some time reflecting on your values, make a list of things you love and a list of things you despise. Doing what you love, within reason, helps overcome fatigue. Eliminating things you despise helps simplify, and simplifying restores energy. Of course, paring down loathings can be a problem since some tasks, like taking out the garbage, must be done. You may be able to recruit help with onerous tasks (for instance, learning how to keep house is good for children). You may find other items on your "hate" list that can also be dispersed, and this will decrease your fatigue.

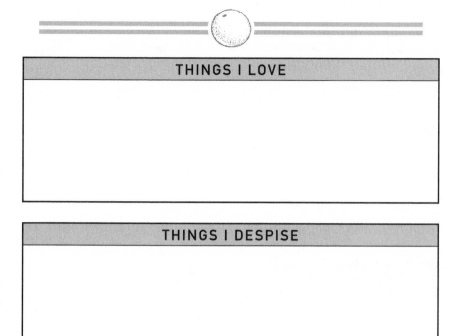

THINGS I LOVE

THINGS I DESPISE

Experience

Experience provides tools you can use for the rest of your life. It helps remedy fatigue only if you bring it to mind, however. Recalling your experiences, you can recognize your strong points and your weak spots. You may set some learning agendas; you may get a better sense of your motivation and others'.

Relax and think back to three significant experiences in your life that jostled or catapulted you in a new direction. They don't have to be the biggest transitions, just significant ones. They may be associated with relationships, ceremonies, school, work, emotions, geography, or health. The transitions may have been positive or negative; they may have been chosen by you or imposed upon you. Keeping in mind that what helped or didn't help in the past is likely to do so again. This includes people.

TRANSITIONAL EXPERIENCES	
What helped?	
Experience #1	
Experience #2	
Experience #3	
What was difficult?	
Experience #1	
Experience #2	
Experience #3	

Capturing Reflections

Take a moment to preserve your reflections before they fly away or evaporate. Just think of what has come to your mind—your good things, your passions, your transitions and more. In your quiet times, you may have decided to do some exploring. You may have made major discoveries or started to shape some new ideas. This is the time to save and savor your excitement.

This is not the time to make lists of pros and cons. Good choices are as much poetry as they are science. Your instincts are as likely to help you make good decisions as is your intellect. The problem is that the more training you get, the more you dismiss your gut—but you can resist. Sue Wilson, an obstetrician and gynecologist, wasn't sure why she kept checking on one new mother who had just delivered a baby. Sue just felt uneasy. She visited and revisited her patient's bedside, checking the vital signs and examining her. The young woman was content and a bit drowsy, as expected. On her last visit, Sue found her patient pale, with a weak and racing pulse and a tense abdomen. It turned out that during the delivery, the woman's uterus had ruptured into her pelvis. Sue's instincts had told her that something was wrong. She paid attention to them, rushed the patient to surgery, and saved her life.

While you are paying attention to your own feelings and instincts, take this opportunity to write about your reflections in your reflection notebook.

Letting Go

To move forward, you will need to release some things. This may be uncomfortable, but remember, if jugglers didn't let go, the show would be over before it started.

Letting go may not be instinctive if you like to fix and control things. You may be reluctant to risk losing power or influence, or you may think that no one else could do the job as well as you. But letting go can actually generate energy, because it will give you more time for what matters. Dispensing with hurtful emotions, attitudes, and schedules frees you to fly.

Use the worksheet below to list the things that you could let go—and who could help you with them.

CAN I LET GO OF ANYTHING?

CAN SOMEONE ELSE AT HOME, WORK, OR IN THE NEIGHBORHOOD TAKE ON A TASK OR TWO?	
Name	Could do what?

Reflection and releasing responsibilities will get you open and ready for the next step: conversation.

STEP THREE: CONVERSATION

What does conversation do for you? You acquire support and feedback, new facts and perspectives. You have less isolation, more resilience, and make better decisions. Conversations will get others involved with your fatigue-ducking maneuvers. Don't be too amazed if your conversation companions restore their own energy, health, and life along with you. Renewing spreads from person to person quite regularly. In fact, that's part of the whole idea.

You can get great advice in conversation. Your scope of feelings and wisdom could be enlarged. I've learned about recovering from the death of a child or spouse while talking with friends who are going through those ordeals. After a chat with an observant visitor to a nursing home, I was able to make recommendations to improve patients' care.

Ground Rules for Good Conversations

If conversations hold such promise of inspiration and caution, what actually goes into a worthy one? For one thing, a conversation is not a rant, speech, or argument. "Conversation" is a particularly delicious word. *Con* means "with" and *versus* means "turn." When you enter a conversation, you are willing to "turn with" one another. Former *British Medical Journal* editor Richard Smith introduced me to an entire book on conversation called, appropriately enough, *Conversation*. Its author, Theodore Zeldin, defines the term like this:

> Conversation is a meeting of minds with different memories and habits. When minds meet, they don't

just exchange facts; they transform them, reshape them, draw different implications from them, and engage in new trains of thought. Conversation doesn't just reshuffle the cards; it creates new cards.

A friend added a down-to-earth comment: "Conversations remind me that I'm not alone or crazy."

Good conversations follow some ground rules:

To start with, have an *open mind and an open heart*; you don't even need to be like-minded. A good conversation needs to be held *in confidence,* so that people feel safe. *Limit complaining.* Nagging issues may need to be aired in order to relieve pressure—but if they dominate, gloom and anger win. *Tell the truth.* You do not need to tell everything, but you do need to be honest. This builds trust. *Listen carefully* because it shows respect. When people are shy, distracted, or tired, they may need to be given *open space* or a bit of prodding. Strangely enough, *silence* can also help conversations. It may be uncomfortable, but silence allows thoughts to emerge and clarify.

Conversation Partners

Conversations usually take place between people who have some sort of relationship, although there are plenty of opportunities to have meaningful conversations with strangers. Having good, deep chats leads to good, deep relationships and *vice versa.* Perhaps one explanation for the bereavement effect—the increased risk of illness and death after a partner's hospitalization or death—is that the remaining person has no one to talk with.

With whom would you like to have a tête-à-tête: A dependable friend? A child? A brother, parent, or aunt? Someone you work out with? A colleague? A mentor? You want to talk with people who don't mind hearing you tell the same story over and over again;

people who share your inner sanctums and are honest with you. People who challenge you or make you feel safe because you know they'll stick around when you are in trouble or sad.

STEP FOUR: PLAN-AND-ACT

The purpose of this last step is to regenerate, to divest yourself of what is dragging you down, and to start fresh. John Gardner called it re-potting. Another gardener I know says, "Right plant, right pot. That's it!" Sometimes you need to move plants and pots around. I know that's not always easy, but I'm going to help you do it.

The first tip is to break things down into small steps. It is best to take them one after the other, but occasional side steps do happen. Taking small steps is smart, not cowardly.

- You can gather allies.
- You build your reputation.
- You gain confidence.
- It is easier to make small adjustments than big ones.
- On occasion, the small steps alone can banish fatigue. For instance, you may not need to change your career but change emphasis.

Two other actions make this last step in the Fatigue Prescription more manageable. One is to simplify and the other is to get organized—at least a smidgen.

What is there to simplify? The spare keys to cars you've traded in, books you'll never read, stacks and files and rubber bands, anything that's dusty or that you haven't worn for two years, even shoes. All of the unnecessary stuff needs to *go*. The clutter can be actual or virtual, physical or mental.

What can you do about it, short of moving house or office? Figure out what is cluttering your life, and get rid of it. A therapist helped herself get into the right frame of mind by changing the word "clutter" to "garbage" as she saved good articles from journals and recycled the rest. Name it what you will and get it out. Peg Bracken's instruction about leftovers makes a nice ditty for more than just refrigerators: "When in doubt, throw it out!" Others think of recycling stuff as part of the Law of Nature. We collect and harvest, save and enjoy, and then it's time for old things to make way for new.

Although most feel that a totally clean desk is a sign of a sick mind, a clean*er* desk prepares you for your successful take-off. It gives a sense of peace that brings strength.

To help you out, here are Dr. Susan Johnson's five organizing principles for the office, which can easily be applied to other areas of life:

- *Do it now.* The key is to look at email messages only when you have time to deal with them. Don't skip any.
- *Work from a clear space.* There should be nothing on your desk except a telephone, a computer, an in/out basket, a coffee cup, and the one task/project you are working on at that moment. When you are pressed for time, take everything (except the aforementioned items) and *put them on the floor.*
- *Keep track of* all *your work commitments.* Keep a single list of every task that you cannot complete immediately. When you finish a task, cross it off. When two thirds of the items on the page are crossed off, tear off the page, re-record all the undone items on to the new page, and keep adding.
- *Use a single master calendar.*

- *Plan by the week.* Daily planning leads to frustration. Stay flexible [but] do not over-schedule.

Be gentle with yourself as you start figuring out what needs to be scaled back or tossed. If you need help, call on an objective friend to help you sort and shovel more effectively.

Start small, of course. What needs to go? When? Whom can you ask for assistance?

Once you get underway, clearing out your clutter and getting organized will get easier. You will be pleased to learn how good it feels to have a clean slate.

CHAPTER 5

THE VALUES PROPOSITION

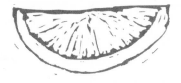

Only to a very limited degree do we strengthen our values by talking about them. Values live or die in every day action.

—John W. Gardner

You might be thinking, "What's the big news? People talk about values all the time." It is true. We are awash in talk of values: family values, cultural values, corporate values, social values, religious values. The problem is, talking isn't the same as listening. Talking isn't the same as doing, either. I recall one of our family's real-life examples: When our daughter Sarah was in high school, she, I, and my husband Jamie were asked to serve on a panel called "Two-Career Families." We figured that Sarah could be the truth squad. We also figured that Sarah had a career as a student, so we changed the panel's title to "A Three-Career Family."

We hadn't given much thought to what made our family work. The panel assignment put our feet to the fire. At our planning caucus, we decided that we relied on three actions: negotiation, accommodation, and recreation. These three actions were based on one underlying conviction: respect. Respect made us able to listen to one another, cut one another some slack, pay attention, forgive, and chuckle. That conviction, in turn, relied on one concept: family first. This fundamental value—not that we called it that—defined our days and nights and set our priorities.

How did this work in real time?

Neither Jamie nor I wanted the other to be the lead parent, so, for example, we went to parent/teachers meetings together. That took some scheduling. When our responsibilities competed with celebrations, we extended birthdays and holiday periods to days or weeks in length. We sent holiday cards after the New Year (in March) to give ourselves a break in December.

We knew that some disapproved of our lives. They said that mothers should be home; fathers shouldn't do the dishes or wash the clothes; and children should have a brother or sister. But I love my work and would have been institutionalized without it. Jamie likes housework, except after some parties when people stay really late. And Hazel Giacomino loved and cared for Sarah from her infancy through eighth grade (and still). We decided to have one child because we wanted to do as much as we could as well as we could, and we knew that we had to set difficult limits. We made it through, too, because we had support from both sets of parents and from friends. One friend carpooled four days a week even though I could reciprocate only on my single "day away" from the hospital. She said, "Women have got to help each other." We were blessed.

Our "Three-Career Family" preparation brought us an awareness of our values so we could think and reflect on them, converse (and negotiate) about them, and schedule our lives to fit them.

We had an unexpected bonus. We not only saw that our goals

were in concert; we discovered that we each believed that the other two had expanded our individual ability to meet our own personal goals. We amplified one another. We served one another. Each of us helped make one another bigger and better, able to accomplish more, discover and learn more, serve the world more.

Looking back, I realize that we needed some courage to go against the grain. It seemed as if we had to give it a good go, however, and we really had no choice. We made it work, keeping our values at the forefront of our lives.

VALUES AND FATIGUE

How do values pertain to recovering from fatigue? Simply this: when you know your deepest commitments, you can make decisions that are in accord with them. You can shed the extras and zero in on what makes your heart soar. The unrestrained quest for balance that puts you in perpetual teeter-totter mode changes completely when you make your values your anchors. Tied to your anchors, your choices are fewer—yet firmer.

Knowing your values is crucial to every step of the Fatigue Prescription: awareness, reflection, conversation, and plan-and-act. Awareness of your values leads to reflection. Reflection about issues, beliefs, feelings, and choices helps you strengthen your values. Understanding your values leads to conversations. Conversations help you hatch plans around them. Plans become action.

Values and priorities shift as your experience and perspective shift. When Sarah was born, the commitment that Jamie and I had to our profession expanded. Sarah came first. Medicine remained a top value; we just adjusted the way we pursued it.

This chapter offers opportunities to recall, define, and affirm your value anchors, to reconstruct your framework. You will see what values can do. You will be able to consider your current values by visiting your memories, your work, and your friends and relatives near and far. Most importantly, you will learn how to leap tall buildings and actually live your values. The goal is to reclaim your heart.

Your values are what matter most to you, a convergence of Stephen Covey's "true north" and "first things first." They are the line you will not cross. They are your foundation and support, the inner guides that direct your behavior—when you are in touch with them.

The whir of the fast lane or the onset of treacherous fatigue can separate you from your values. That is unfortunate because values inform your judgment about what is right and wrong, good or ill. They motivate you and are the mainspring of your fulfillment and joy. They are the basis of the meaning *in* your life. Values are the beliefs you won't give up no matter what. Your values determine the way you act when no one is looking. When shared, values hold families, organizations, and societies together.

HOW VALUES WORK

You see values operating in families, schools, churches, and clubs. Parents, relatives, teachers, and leaders are all carriers of values. Companies demonstrate their values via their codes of ethics, colleges via their honor codes, and the military via its rules. Values are more often caught than taught.

For example, as life happens, you are touched by *kindness*—and want to pass it on. You respect those who have *integrity*—and decide to practice it. You enjoy the research, learning, and innovation that go into being highly regarded, so you seek *excellence*, despite its demands. You find that *trust* makes it easier to address challenges. You discover that *mutual openness and shared interests* can grow into friendship, even love. *Respect* helps build strong communities. You appreciate *fairness* and *justice*, especially when you have empathy for or inhabit low places. And so you learn and choose your values.

Putting values to work makes your life more fulfilling and easier. Values transform beliefs into ideas, ideas into words, and words into actions. Dr. Christine Einert, a pioneer in occupational health, had the unalterable conviction that workers should not have to sacrifice their health in order to earn a living. Statistics and observation led her to suspect that short-handled hoes contributed to farm laborers' back problems. She decided to work alongside the field-hands who used those hoes to tend crops in the blistering farmlands of central California. Dr. Einert was able to document physical problems associated with using these hoes, and with persistence and support, her recommendations led to eliminating the implement that the workers called El Diablo. By applying her values, she was able to help cause a remarkable improvement in worker health.

A values list can be a tickler file. We all need reminders to recall important things, but fatigue can erase values like waves taking down a sand castle. Will you rush off to the next meeting or pause to hug a colleague whose father just died? Are you so absorbed in your own daily grind that you ignore others affected by the most recent earthquake or plague? Do you value yourself enough to take care of yourself? Your values help you to do the things you believe in, but you have to be aware enough to get the point.

Decisions rooted in values gain muscle. When schedules reflect values, time magically appears. If "family" matters, creating togetherness with vacations, long weekends, meals, telephone, or instant messaging all becomes habit. If friendship and health are both essential, friends or colleagues can talk and walk at the same time.

Values are the basis of your pleasure when you live them. Not that living values is always easy. Sometimes you forego one pleasure for another. One father who re-arranged his schedule to spend more time with his family gave up some income in the process. He said, "I'm doing great! Sure I lost a little bit of money, but I would *pay* to be this happy! I'm married, parenting, and exercising!" He had regained his meaning in life and his joy.

It's not always easy, of course. Values can collide with each other or be difficult to live. When work and fatigue overwhelm you, finishing the to-do list may seem your most important value.

This is why understanding what your *real* values are is so central to the Fatigue Prescription. As you become aware of your ideals, you can reflect upon and sort them, have conversations about them, and then plan-and-act to become what you most want to be—in good health and with energy left over.

THE COMPANY YOU KEEP

Older or younger, friend, colleague, or stranger, the people around you can contribute to your values quest and renewing campaign. You will likely find that you define the people around you by their actions, which, in turn, depend on their values. It is no shock that others ascertain or think they ascertain your values by observing you. Here are some ways to appraise the values of others that I have distilled from years of RENEW workshops.

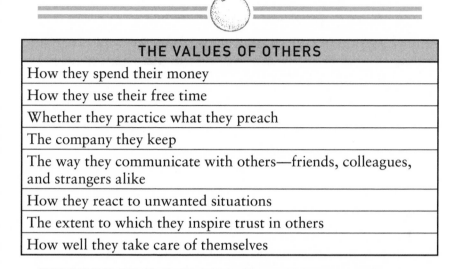

THE VALUES OF OTHERS
How they spend their money
How they use their free time
Whether they practice what they preach
The company they keep
The way they communicate with others—friends, colleagues, and strangers alike
How they react to unwanted situations
The extent to which they inspire trust in others
How well they take care of themselves

RECALLING AND REVISING YOUR OWN VALUES

Waking up from your fatigue and getting your priorities straight again means reclaiming your own values. How do you do it?

"It's always best to start at the beginning," Glinda told Dorothy in *The Wizard of Oz*. The beginning in this case is likely to be your deepest beliefs and convictions, the ones that you absorbed at a young age, at home, in your place of worship, or at school.

I know I caught values early on. I vividly recall conversations about community-mindedness, learning, deference to elders, and self-sufficiency. I also absorbed the message of caring for others. Perhaps that's why I became a doctor.

Take a breath and get ready; stretch your body and mind, and think way back and way deep. What are some of your earliest values?

MY EARLY VALUES
Values gained at home:
Values gained from religion/moral/spiritual training:
Values gained at school:

Take a good look at your list. Do those values still resonate? Maybe some and not others? That's ok! Values aren't static. They may take years or just a minute to change.

You are altered by events and observations that shift your values. You start off, have gains and setbacks, start again, grow ill and then get better, win the lottery, or lose loved ones. Values that you once held firm may wash out as others come in. Some of the old ones persist, of course, brighter and more powerful than when you were growing up.

I still have most of my early values. Faith has grown in importance as I faced desolate times. Complete independence and self-sufficiency, on the other hand, have become less important to me as I savor friendships and rely more on others.

I have added some values over the years, too. I hold neighborhood health and the health of the environment as higher values than I did before, for example.

What about you? Have you misplaced, dropped, or downsized some values? Why? Have you added some central principles over the years? What was your impetus?

Compare and Contrast

Should the values held by others influence the values you hold? Should it matter what other people think about your values? Not really, but you live in a particular time and place and are part of a particular culture. Understanding where and how your values match—or depart from—those around you can help you understand your own values and test your commitment to them.

The values in the following chart are compiled from hundreds of RENEW sessions. Over and over, these are the values that lead the pack. Some of yours will likely match these. This will give you some sense of the universal values in your time and place. Some of your values may be quite different from these. This will give you some sense of your uniqueness.

You have some choices about looking at the Values Priority table. You may want to cut to the chase and look at the column with the rankings. *But wait!* If you like puzzles and want more of a challenge, you could try playing a "game" with the Values Priority table. One big advantage of playing the game is that you record results of conversations with your family and friends about their values, too. This is a significant element in taking your next renewing steps.

First, cover the column at the far right. (The list is in random order.) Try, try not to peek.

Then read the values list.

In the second column on the left, write down your own ranking of each value, from 1 to 14 (with 1 being the highest ranking). You may have ties in your list and that's all right.

Now write the rankings you discovered from your family and friends.

Finally, uncover the right hand column and see how those stack up compared to the wider world, represented here by RENEW participants. (The RENEW rankings include some ties, so there are repeated numbers.)

THE VALUES PRIORITY TABLE			
Values	Your Own Ranking	Ranking of Others	
		Your Friends and Family	RENEW-ers Ranking
Respect (for self and others)			6
Noble goals (caring, altruism, giving back)			5
Family			2
Self (esteem, worth, love, fulfill-ment)			2
How the world should work (truth, ethics, freedom)			8
Peace of mind/state of being (opti-mism, flexibility, serenity)			5
Honesty/integrity			1
Wonder/mystery/higher power			8
Compassion/kindness/empathy/trust			3
Joy/happiness			9
How to act toward others (gener-osity. appreciation, openness)			4
How to work with others (team, sharing, reliability)			4
Learning and knowledge			7
Love			9

YOUR CURRENT VALUES

You've looked at the values you grew up with and the values you've discarded and added along the way. You've tested them against others' values, and you have an idea of what matters most to you.

Pour a cuppa, scratch what itches, shoo away what is bugging you (in person or on your mind), and fill in this chart. Write your values. Let go; cut loose! Heck, *draw* the values; put them in color. Use crayons, or inks, or paints! That is how your brain works best, by coalescing input from several neuro-physiological pathways and using both your right and left hemispheres.

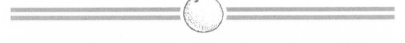

MY VALUES
I will not give these up, no matter what. These are my convictions. They compel, propel, and fulfill me.

Do whatever it takes to keep yourself constantly reminded of your values. Say them out loud. Say them to someone else. Hearing yourself helps declare their truth and importance and also helps your memory. Laminate your values on a card and put it in your wallet. Stick them to the refrigerator door, the bathroom mirror, your office bulletin board. Convert them to a screensaver. A nurse told me how she remembers hers: "We have to change our email password every three months, so I go to my list of values and choose one. I'm on 'forgiveness' right now." Another nurse hangs a picture of her family on the lanyard around her neck along with her ID.

Values are the framework for setting your priorities in life. They form the launch pad for waking up from your fatigue and regaining your purpose. Carry your values in your mind and heart, silently or aloud. Listen to them, because *you are your values*. Let your beliefs hold you fast. Stay anchored to them. This is the best way to free yourself from fatigue—and to stay free.

CHAPTER 6

DISCOVERING WHAT YOU REALLY WANT AND HOW TO GET IT

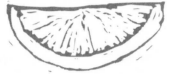

There's nothing wrong with searching for happiness, but...what gives far greater comfort to the soul is meaning..."

—Sir Laurens van der Post

You are well on your way to leaving fatigue behind. You have already done the groundwork. This chapter sees you well on your way to filling the Fatigue Prescription. It will help you think about success, because knowing your own definition of success gives you one yardstick to measure whether you are living your values. I will go into detail about ways to make changes because change is a bugaboo for many and yet it is coming. Excellence is on the agenda, too, because it is controversial yet worth considering. I will again mention "Encouragers," because they can get you started and help you over humps to the finish. Since you still have some miles to cover, I will remind you to take care of yourself, to be kind, and to dream. Prudence, courage, resilience, and commitment will round out your supplies for your fatigue-defeating campaign: *prudence* because it helps you take reasonable chances, *courage* because you need it to put your face into the wind, *resilience* because inevitably something will go amiss, and *commitment* because it adds steel to your purpose and is a shield against distraction.

By the end of the chapter, as your fatigue continues to recede, you will discover dreams and goals that are replenished or new. You will also have polished connections with key people and with your own qualities and commitments. You can sketch a rough plan for supplanting your fatigue with things that really matter.

WHAT DO YOU REALLY WANT?

I would like to add a cautionary note before you continue this adventure: It may not be wise to set a definite goal. The world is big and has many needs and opportunities. You may even decide to tackle the unachievable. That's all right, for, as the theologian Reinhold Niebuhr said, "Nothing that is worth doing can be achieved in our lifetime..." You'll want to have some flexibility in considering your destiny.

Success

Your quest for success should be more about "want to" than "ought to." You can get exhausted running on someone else's treadmill. Being successful has more to do with your own wisdom and longings than anyone else's expectations of you.

You may interpret success in kaleidoscopic ways. If you look back at the Renew-O-Meter, you may get some ideas about what you consider success so far. Another way to reflect on your feelings regarding success is to learn how others define it. In March 2009, the Harris Poll (at the request of Age Wave, a company known for age-related research and communications) conducted a national survey of 2,000 people who ranged in age from 21 to 84, asking "How do you define success?" Here are their results:

- Having a loving family and friends (51–69 percent)
- The freedom to do what I want (37 percent)
- Achieving financial independence (33 percent)
- Having inner peace (30 percent)
- Being true to myself and not selling out (19 percent)
- Having power and influence (3 percent)

A group of physician-leaders came up with the following definitions:

- Achieving goals
- Enjoying good relations with family
- Having the time to do what you want to do
- Feeling happiness and contentment
- Living in harmony with your values
- Making a difference in someone's life
- Balancing service with hedonism
- Seeing success in those you nurture—children, students, colleagues

My husband Jamie added, "The number of people who will pray for you when you need it." John Gardner said, "Being an example of God's handiwork." And a classmate added, "Going to my high school reunion even though I looked a mess."

Go through these lists and circle or star the definitions of success that make the most sense to you. It is likely that some of your fatigue is related to pushing automatically for success in ways that aren't very important to you. Defining your idea of success will help you re-sort your priorities according to your values.

Despite the attraction of these aims, your pursuit of success on your own terms can put you in hot water. A group of health care workers pointed out some of the adverse consequences of success:

- Others' jealousy
- Divisions within groups
- Destroyed friendships
- Becoming distant from family members who haven't "achieved"
- Losing support of those who had other goals for you
- Loss of freedom—being successful may make you the go-to person, which is limiting when people "go-to" you all the time

You may have experienced some of this pain. Think about whether the price of success—or the way you are going after it—is too high. This may very well affect your plans.

Once you've decided, ask yourself what you think it will take for you to accomplish what you most fervently want. Your growth, happiness, and therefore your success may depend upon this. Here are some ways you might start. There is space at the bottom to add your ideas.

- Regroup with important people, including family, friends, and allies
- Stick with the things you set out to do
- Relax and smile
- Change directions
- Change jobs
- Speak up
- Settle down

- Take a break
- Open up

_____

_____

_____

_____

Going for Excellence—or Is Good Enough Really Good Enough?
As you push back against the fatigue that is gnawing at you, you face a prevalent and nagging dilemma: Do I set my sights on excellence or do I just try to get by? Should I go for the gold or settle for making it to the try-outs?

"Satisfactory" may be as good as it gets in some circumstances. There is no doubt that it is a victory merely to survive some crushing days and wretched years. Treading water is better than sinking.

The fact is, "good enough" and "satisfactory" won't get anyone to the far galaxies, however. And we need and want to go there. It is also true that you can't be excellent at everything, so you will need to set priorities not only about *what* you do, but *how well* you do it. Your decisions will depend on your inclinations, energy, intellect, and, above all, your values. Refining your priorities and standards can help you fill the Fatigue Prescription and head you toward excellence.

HOW TO GET WHAT YOU REALLY WANT

You've taken a look at success and its pros and cons. You've reflected about your preferred standard of excellence. You've documented how you spend your time and how you wish you could spend it. Now you are ready to start setting your post-fatigue priorities.

What Goes into Making Changes?

Back in Chapter 4 you looked at your life and things you may want to change—where you might like to go, a safety net, what you would like to learn. As your fatigue wanes and your energy rises, the bright light on the horizon is change.

You certainly are not alone if you have conflicting sentiments about making some changes. There isn't much of an alternative if you want to get out of the doldrums. As Alcoholics Anonymous points out, "Insanity is doing the same thing over and over and each time expecting different results."

A few years ago the Values Action Committee, a multidisciplinary Conversation Group© that met for several years at California Pacific Medical Center, made some observations about change:

- Change is multidimensional. It is both welcome and unwelcome. It creates opportunity.
- Change involves power—my power to work with it and others' power over me.
- Resistance is huge when change hits without warning.
- Accepting things I can't change is not the same as just going with the flow. Acceptance takes some thought.
- Change can be uncomfortable, but it puts me in a state of awareness, ready to go.
- Changing requires energy!
- Making the decision to change is not always a lightning-bolt event.
- Change affects everyone. If the change is at work, it affects my family, too.
- Change can be positive and exciting.

These comments show the tangle of good news and bad news that doing something new can entail. Businessman Harvey Mackay outlined some of the difficulties with change:

> Even when change is elective, it will disorient you. You may go through anxiety. You will miss aspects of your former life...The trick is to know in advance...that you're going to be thrown off your feet by it. So you prepare for this inevitable disorientation and steady yourself to get through it. Then you take the challenge, make the change, and achieve your dreams.

Some of our understanding about making adjustments comes from studies of patients who have been advised to alter their lives for medical reasons. See if these change-avoiding "methods" fit you. You may not understand why you need to change. Or you just might not want to change, no matter how imperative it is that you do so, like the alcoholic who told me, "Doc, I know the booze is killing me, but I like how it feels!" Sometimes you may feel that you don't have enough information, or that there are too many competing messages about how and why to change. You may not feel you are worth the trouble—a terrible consequence of low self-esteem or depression. Finally, it is quite common to make light of change. You may think that giving up a cherished behavior will be simple, but you may overestimate your will power or your "won't power."

The important thing is finding a way to overcome your resistance to change and understanding how change will happen. Frequently there is a six-stage path to change:

1. Pre-contemplation: "Never! Go away. Get outta here. Not my problem. Not my cup of tea."
2. Contemplation: "Well, maybe. I'll give it some thought."
3. Preparation: "I'll line up some help."
4. Action: "I am actually making the change."
5. Maintenance: "I can do this, I'm feeling better...but I need to strengthen my resolve so I don't drift."
6. Relapse: "I slipped back into my old ways. This is hard!" "Relapse" isn't the end game, and self-flagellation doesn't help. Your internal chat could go like this, "I didn't make it this time, but at least I learned something. If I made progress before, I can do it again—and I'll figure out better ways."

Barriers to Change

For many, *fear* is in the forefront of barriers to moving ahead. Fear comes in many flavors.

- *Fear of failure*: "All that effort for what? I don't want to wind up disappointing others or myself."
- *Fear of the unknown*: "I don't feel comfortable without a map. I dread wandering around lost. What will happen if I make this change?"
- *Fear of loss*: "Loss" could mean loss of reputation, relationships, self-esteem, public standing, identity, or values.
- *Fear of success*: You may not see yourself as being "successful" or deserving of success. Success seems as if it requires more work to maintain than the status quo. You may be scared of what you will do with success should you attain it.
- *Fear of the outcome*: You might go broke. You might become overwhelmed.

- *Fear of being judged:* By society, your spouse or partner, a boss, or even strangers.
- *Fear of getting in trouble.*
- What fears prevent *you* from moving ahead?

_____

_____

_____

_____

_____

_____

_____

Just as fears are barriers to change, so are "not enoughs": insufficient time, energy, money, information, or self-esteem or a lack of impetus or encouragement. Your own attitudes could also be a hurdle. If you can't believe in the possibility of a positive outcome, why bother with hope? If it just doesn't seem likely that change could make your dreams come true, why bother to try?

Of course, the flip side of "not enough" is too much. The fatigue from overwork or from being tired of it all may prove to be a barrier to change. Too much comfort can lead to inertia and an aversion to risk. Over-analysis may lead you to paralysis, or to bury your energy in trivial and circular reasoning. Too much clutter and busyness can also hinder moving forward. The workload itself can be crushing. Anger can blur your vision. Martyrdom—choosing to suffer or to be a victim—can poison your progress because having excuses is easier than changing.

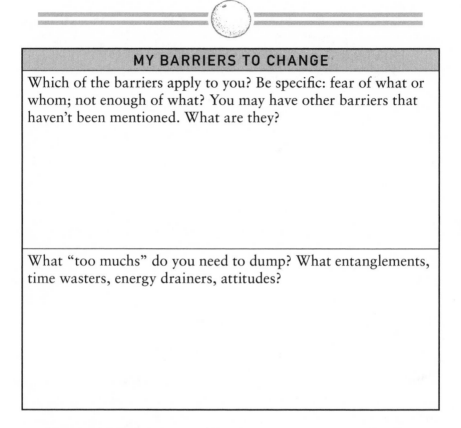

MY BARRIERS TO CHANGE

Which of the barriers apply to you? Be specific: fear of what or whom; not enough of what? You may have other barriers that haven't been mentioned. What are they?

What "too muchs" do you need to dump? What entanglements, time wasters, energy drainers, attitudes?

Once you understand your own particular barriers, you can decide how to work on them. That is a good choice.

Boosters to Change

What motivates you to get out of your muck or rut or comfort zone? What propels you into exciting possibilities? Some say that barriers can themselves be boosters: fear, fatigue, finances, and threats of loss. Sometimes you change because you can't stand the anguish, heartbreak, injustice, or punishment any more. A friend of mine finally left her marriage when her husband deliberately broke her leg by hitting her with the car.

Others favor the vision and the pull of positives. You may change because you are determined to follow your calling, to reach your definition of success, to be happy, or to be "better." This increases your sense of self-worth. That, in itself, is an incentive to change, because, frankly, you admire yourself when you take on something new. Seeing a glimmer of hope or curiosity can push you forward.

Some people are motivated by holding themselves accountable. A successful change agent who led a corporate reorganization said, "I had no choice. It was my idea. I had my pride and honor to uphold."

Change may start or accelerate when priorities or situations evolve. Children come along, parents' health declines, or you move from one town to another, so living arrangements, budgets, and even chores turn topsy-turvy.

Boosting Your Boosters

Behavior modification experts have found several simple yet powerful ways to help you make changes. One is to put a rubber band around your wrist and give it a good snap when you want another chocolate truffle, tumble into a spiral of downward thinking, or find yourself watching TV deep into the night. This will give yourself a physical jolt that can divert you from temptation into a more productive vein. Several other suggestions came up at a RENEW workshop on rituals. Bill Stewart, the physician who heads CPMC's Institute for Health and Healing, said at a RENEW conference, "Every day is starting over. You have a 15-second interval to make a change, to get up, move around and make a decision before you sink back into your usual." Jamie said, "But you have to decide what is your first priority." Psychiatrist

Jean Shinoda Bolen added, "Breaking a habit gets easier. You may be able to do it yourself or you may need a run buddy or a circle of friends. When you say your intention to witnesses, it provides motivation and energy."

Finding Your Encouragers

One of the biggest boosters to change is having help: good parents, brothers, sisters, aunts, uncles, cousins, colleagues, mentors, and friends. They are some of the best creatures on earth. They are the Encouragers. Encouragers put courage—their heart—into you. Their version of the mantra from *The Little Engine That Could* is, "I think *you* can. I think *you* can. I think *you* can." Or even "I *know* you can. I *know* you can. I *know* you can."

My parents were Encouragers supreme. As we discussed my dream of becoming a physician, they were unfailingly positive, and they even found me a role model, a rare young woman physician, who answered my questions and showed me that my aspiration could come true.

Strangers can be Encouragers, too. Anyone who helps an elder across the street, lends a hand when you are struggling with the gas pump, or even smiles and tells you to have a nice day is an Encourager, often just when you need it most.

Think about who or what has been a bright light to you, a booster, an Encourager. Who has said "Go for it"? What situations have prodded you to move ahead? Are you one of the people who can say, "Getting fired was the best thing that ever happened to me"? Take your time. Use extra space if you need it. Be prepared to be surprised, perhaps warmed, by your answers.

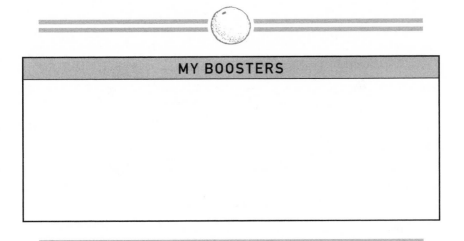

MY BOOSTERS

Now let's look inside. What are your assets, your own reservoir of talents, attitudes, and passions that, when tapped into, can move you forward? This should be a long list and will likely take awhile to complete. It should make you smile, as you discover some of your internal treasures.

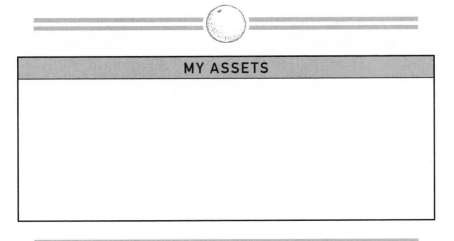

MY ASSETS

YOUR OWN STOCKPILE FOR RENEWING

Along with knowing your own special barriers, boosters, and behavior modification techniques, it would be smart to have a supply of just a few other qualities and practices to help you on your fatigue-conquering quest.

Prudence

I would like to champion *prudence* as a life- and reputation-saving virtue. It is the look before you leap. It is the ten-second pause before you fly off the handle. It is reading the outraged email once more before you hit "send."

Being prudent doesn't interrupt your momentum; it helps you find your safest and surest way. In your search-and-recovery operation for defeating fatigue, you likely will come upon unexpected and unwanted hazards. Taking reasonable risks will be part of the adventure. When you're ready, you can take some chances, picking your steps carefully as you go.

To make your life better and rid yourself of fatigue, you will need to take risks, but look ahead prudently and give yourself the reassurance of Plans B, C, and maybe D. It's akin to having cab fare to get you home just in case the date goes sour. Or planning before ending a deadening marriage, as a friend of mine did. She took several years to develop financial, managerial, and organizational skills as a volunteer so she could later support herself and her kids.

Taking Care

When you get right down to it, all you have is yourself. That is why it is not selfish to take care of yourself. Yes, I believe that self-sacrifice is often necessary. But if you work yourself to ashes there is nothing left with which to ignite the rest of your life.

One of the best ways to take care of yourself is to be gentle with yourself, especially when you are taking risks or undergoing a major change. Congratulate yourself, even out loud. Write "xo" notes to yourself and stick them where you will see them. Celebrate your accomplishments! Reward your steps forward! Why not get a massage, watch a movie, eat a succulent peach, hike a new trail, or paint some pictures? The celebration and reward can be relaxing, and when you are relaxed it's easier to work hard.

For so many people, being self-critical comes naturally. You try to be perfect but can't be, so anger and self-doubt bubble up, especially when you feel criticized. Part of taking care of yourself is choosing to stop that negative thinking. Go back to snapping that rubber band around your wrist. Above all, do not compromise your health—physical or mental. Remember, you are all you have.

WAYS TO TAKE CARE OF YOURSELF
Some thoughtful young physicians offered these good-natured suggestions for being considerate to yourself:
Keep playing with kids before you forget what it was like to be one.
Stop competing with others and live within your means.
Manage time rather than letting time manage you.
Take advantage of every opportunity, especially with regard to experience and learning.
Travel
Give yourself some credit.
Don't delay your life while you're working toward your goal.
Quit your job if it's killing you.
Get some sleep.

WAYS TO TAKE CARE OF YOURSELF
Get help with cleaning the house.
Ask, "Is this really necessary?"
Marry the right person and be nice to him or her.
Read for pleasure.
Think often, "Will this matter a year from now; ten years from now?" and then act accordingly.

Dreams

Dreams are another essential item in your renewing stockpile. You can dream for the near future or the faraway. Dreams are especially important if you feel as if you are losing ground. Or if your goals seem too monumental or insurmountable. Or if getting through the Fatigue Prescription seems beyond you. Others have walked in your shoes. They say to keep on dreaming, as did Langston Hughes:

DREAMS

Hold fast to dreams.
For if dreams die
life is a broken-winged bird
that cannot fly.
Hold fast to dreams.
For when dreams go
life is a barren field
frozen with snow.

You could dream about anything. What would be your perfect job? Where would you really like to live? How do you wish you could spend your time? And how would you really *not* like to spend your time? These are pretty straightforward dreams, which is good, because they are easy to remember and they are motivating.

Cultural anthropologist Angeles Arrien takes another tack and gives you permission to *re*-dream. When old dreams flounder or wither, re-dreaming can freshen them or bring new hopes and dreams, and, later, plans. Whether new or refurbished, dreams provide impetus.

Courage

Summoning your own courage is part of getting fatigue down for the count. When you believe in the supreme importance of something—home, friends, doing what's right, self-preservation—and when you name it as a value, you can summon the courage to conduct yourself as you choose.

Courage helps you act despite fear. Courage is there for you, available on the spot and durable. You can use it to make tough choices and to persevere, to conquer your fatigue.

Resilience

Resilience complements courage. It is the ability to bounce back from dashed hopes or disillusionment. Having resilience is like being a good tennis player who awaits a rocket serve with knees flexed, ready to lunge in any direction and slam the ball back. As with courage, resilience is within you, at the ready. How do you know you have it? Think back to the times you recovered after sorrow or disappointment. Although fatigue drains that capability, just as it drains your energy bucket, you can turn on the Fatigue Prescription spigot to refill both.

What can you do to build resilience? How can you foster positive outcomes? You can take a break! Sleep, including a nap, counts as a break. How about nurturing strong and healthy relationships by having a regular date with a friend or partner, or a real vacation without email or text messaging? You can take a vacation from the news. You can swim, walk, or run. You could play the zither, pray or meditate, write a poem, or make friends with a baby. Along the way, stop chewing over regrets.

You could also raise your resilience by giving up control and settling for influence. You cannot command the waves, but you can still keep your hand on the tiller. This shift saves energy and helps open vistas toward which way to bounce.

Finally, you can change your perspective. I met an engineer who was recently diagnosed with multiple sclerosis. He was actually glad to learn what had been causing his left leg weakness. He can't ride a bike anymore, but he's relieved he can walk. He thinks of his good leg as a helper and doesn't consider his other leg "bad." When my classmate broke her ankle while on vacation, she said, "Well, it was on the last day of the trip. The empty seats on the plane let me stretch out. The doctor in Mexico made a house call, and I got lots of attention from strong, handsome men." How bad can that be? How resilient!

Commitment
The final essential supply for your anti-fatigue campaign is commitment. This means going beyond *pledging* to *doing*. Whether in marriage vows, professional oaths, or determining to take a new direction, you may find yourself wavering. Psychologist Rollo May said that's all right: "The relationship between commitment and doubt is [not] an antagonistic one. Commitment is healthiest when it is not without doubt but in spite of doubt." Harnessing

the doubt and making the commitment puts the Force, your force, with you.

One of my favorite observations about commitment comes from an adventure book published in 1951. W.H. Murray, in *The Scottish Himalayan Expedition*, describes some hiking friends' uncertainties and vacillations that finally crystallized into action, allowing Scotland's pioneering climbers to blaze the way for the conquest of Everest.

> Until one is committed there is always hesitancy, the chance to draw back, always ineffectiveness...the moment one definitely commits oneself, then Providence moves too...A whole stream of events issues from the decision, [bringing] all manner of unforeseen accidents and meetings and material assistance which no [one] could have dreamed would come his way.

He ended by quoting Goethe:

> Whatever you can do or dream you can, begin it
> Boldness has genius, power, and magic in it.

Now it is your time to bring some magic into your life and to start your own healing. In the worksheet on the next page, consider your commitments as a countdown: 5, 4, 3, 2, 1, and lift off!

MY COMMITMENTS

In the next five *weeks I will start to build/rebuild my network. Here are family, friends, mentors, and allies I will contact:*

Name	Contact Info

I will learn something new in four *categories:*

Category	Subject
Home life	
Work	
Civic affairs	
For myself	

I will celebrate three *things:*

What to Celebrate	How

I will stop two *things:*

What to Stop	How

MY COMMITMENTS

I make the following one *commitment based on my values:*

CHAPTER 7

GET IN SHAPE

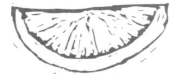

One ought, everyday at least, to hear a little song, read a good poem, see a fine picture, and, if it were possible, to speak a few reasonable words.

—Johann von Goethe

Ever been on one of those expeditions where you trek or cycle over mountains or paddle rushing waterways? The outfitters or sponsors of the events assure you that you will enjoy the experience more and are less likely to drop out or get hurt if you are in good shape. Ditto with fatigue. If you start out fit, you're better able to deal fatigue a blow when it threatens; you're less likely to drop out or get hurt.

To be fatigue-fit, you need to be buff in five areas of your life: your personal relationships, your spirituality, your physical health, your work, and your attitude. Here's what I mean:

FATIGUE-FIGHTING FITNESS
Have *strong relationships* with family, friends, colleagues, organizations, and neighborhood.
Have a *spiritual side* or *practice a religion*. These are not mutually exclusive.
Take care of yourself. Be healthy and rested and know how to set limits so you can keep on learning and growing.
Find purpose in your work, whether paid or unpaid. Derive meaning and pleasure from what you do.
Have an *upbeat attitude.* You need to envision grander possibilities and believe that progress is possible.

The following worksheet will help you determine your current level of buffness:

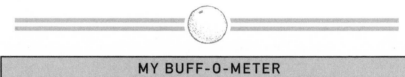

MY BUFF-O-METER
I have strong family, work, and social relationships. ❑ Yes ❑ No
My life has robust spiritual or religious elements. ❑ Yes ❑ No
I take good care of my body. ❑ Yes ❑ No
I enjoy work. ❑ Yes ❑ Mainly ❑ Not really ❑ No
My attitude is generally positive. ❑ Yes ❑ It depends ❑ No

This chapter is all about shaping up. It follows along with the five points in your Buff-O-Meter and ends with ways to fit fitness into your life.

RELATIONSHIPS

Unless you are a hermit, people are part of your life. They are key to the four steps of the Fatigue Prescription: awareness → reflection → conversation → and plan-and-act. People you have relationships with can be mentors, Encouragers, friends, or family. You have an enormous effect on the people around you as well. How contagious is your fatigue?

To be sure, no one is on a high plane all the time. It's unrealistic. On a daily basis, even your own body has peaks and valleys. For example, in response to stimuli from your brain, your cortisol (an energy hormone), peaks in the very early morning, falls during the day, and reaches a low when you are asleep. You may be aware of up and down curves in your relationships, too. Just as with your energy bucket, your connections with others stay robust only with renewing.

SPIRITUALITY AND RELIGION

Almost nothing else can move you or touch you as much as spirituality and religion. San Francisco rabbi Eric Weiss points out that both spirituality and religion entail awe. When you *name* your awe—Adonai, Allah, Jesus, Buddha's way—you define your religion. He adds that religion provides structure, rules, and practices, and may ascribe power to a supreme being; spirituality often involves curiosity, imagination, and the senses. My husband defines three elements of spirituality: reflection, connection, and meaning.

The Fatigue Prescription has you engaged with all of these.

Many people find spirituality, faith, and religion are the foundation of their lives and the reach beyond themselves. Their beliefs are activators and the basis of their enthusiasm. (In Greek, "en" means within; "thus" is from "theo" which means God. So enthusiasm literally means "God within.")

Being connected with your religion or spirituality—your mysteries, joys, and grandeurs—can show you a way out of fatigue.

How do you get in touch with these powers within? Being in an oak grove helped the Druids; medieval cathedrals' stained glass windows helped peasants and nobles alike who worshipped there; bonfires under starry nights provided native peoples the setting for telling stories and passing along traditions. It's not so different nowadays.

Places and ceremonies may open up feelings or impart majesty or peace. The outdoors, beauty, and rituals all can link you to deep truths. You probably know the best place or time or thought to help you to get in touch with your spiritual connections. Your spirit is obtainable and can be at your service. It will be there for you most dependably if you are a willing, open-hearted searcher.

BUILDING YOUR BODY'S STAYING POWER: PHYSICAL FITNESS

You've been paying attention to your relationships and your spirituality. Now it's time to return to your body. In this section I will offer some facts and opinions about food, fitness, medications, supplements, and more to supply you energy and fortitude as you use the Fatigue Prescription.

No one says it is easy to become or stay physically fit. If it were, you wouldn't hear train loads of advice about diet and exercise. I'll keep mine short.

Food and Exercise

Food

- Spices are better for you than salt.
- The brighter a vegetable's color, the more nutritional value it has.
- Calories count—keep them low, diverse, and tasty.
- Using small plates helps make modest servings look heftier.
- Fat has nine calories per gram. Sugars and starches have four calories per gram.
- If you don't burn the calories you eat, they get converted to fat that will pad your frame. Do the math. Fat *in* is more likely to put fat *on* than carbohydrates. Fat cells make and secrete chemicals that cause inflammation inside your arteries. Eventually, the irritated cells in your arteries die and form "gruel" (that's the scientific term!) that collects inside the wall of your arteries. This makes an ever-expanding pillow-shaped obstruction to blood flow. When the pillow gets too full or bursts, your circulation gets cut off and disaster strikes.

Exercise

- Exercise is good for you.
- It can be a bore. Therefore, find exercise you like so you can stick with it. Companions may help.
- Exercise burns calories, builds muscle, and dissolves built-up fats.
- It builds two kinds of muscles in addition to your heart. One kind helps endurance and the other helps your speed and strength.
- Exercise can decrease falls and fractures and increase sleep. Yoga and tai chi count as exercise; and they also help with the stretching that keeps you limber.
- You can start to exercise and get good results at least up to

age 92. That's good because there's an ever-improving chance that you and your elders will live to be over 100 in good health if you take care.

- Your goal should be to exercise a minimum of thirty minutes a day five days a week. The effort should increase your pulse rate by about 50 percent. Check with your doctor before you start a new routine.

Now let's assess your current fitness level.

MY BODY'S STAYING POWER: PHYSICAL FITNESS
How does my weight now compare to my size in high school?
❑ My weight is within 5–10 pounds.
❑ My size has increased by 2–4 levels.
❑ I've gained 10–20 pounds per decade.
❑ I'm not overweight, I'm under-tall.
I strain to keep up with the crowd or am the last one to make it up the stairs because I am out of breath. ❑ Yes ❑ No
For exercise, I:
❑ Do as little as possible, and I like it that way.
❑ Am not proud of my record and I'm thinking about changing it.
❑ Can do just about whatever I want to do, especially if I take a rest along the way.
❑ Lift weights and/or have a regular exercise routine.

Physical fitness can go a long way toward reducing your fatigue. I am a certified exercise hater, but even I was able to learn to do it.

Walking is my exercise of choice because it's easy: it requires no new equipment and no training, and there are some nice trails near our house. Walking became less of an ordeal when I discovered wildflowers along the trails. First I counted them: twenty-three kinds in one day! Then I learned their common and botanical names and how the Miwoks used them. After some weeks, Jamie and I, interested in reclaiming nature, took on The Dell, a shady notch off the trail extending up a hill and choked with highly flammable non-native Scotch broom. We set to work taking out the broom and other weeds. As we worked, we recruited allies and an entire community grew around the project. I formed friendships with walkers who offer good company. The piquant conversations decrease my misery from the exercise that I still hate. We all enjoy the Dell which now has sticky monkey flowers scattered through it, and native grasses grow along its springtime stream. My self-improvement project also meant that I had to cut back on food, even chocolate chip cookies. Along with decreasing butter and having smaller servings, I found that brushing and flossing immediately after dinner were key. I would rather go over Niagara Falls in a barrel than floss my teeth twice in one evening, so flossing eliminated my night-time snacks. Viola! *Twenty-five pounds gone and still gone* (with some wavering), nineteen years ago.

Natural Foods, Supplements, and Drugs

I can understand why "natural" seems to equal "good." Fresh air is better than foul; clean water is better than dirty. If you think about it, however, you can come up with plenty of examples in which "natural" is bad. Poison oak and poison ivy are natural.

Nature is full of minerals that don't do our bodies any good, such as asbestos, lead, and mercury. Whereas you do need traces of zinc, but put in the wrong place—your nose—and sometimes with even one dose, you can lose your sense of smell.

Many people approach supplements with the philosophy, "more is better." But if you have reasonable eating habits and are generally healthy, what's to supplement? Your body has been adapted through eons to thrive on good sense and good food. And there are plenty of ways to have too much of different supplements. We know, for example, that too much Vitamin A causes liver, bone, and skin damage. Excess Vitamin D causes kidney stones and other disorders secondary to high calcium. High doses of Vitamin C (over 2000 mg or 2 gm per day) have never been shown to prevent or ease colds for run-of-the mill people like you and me, but does cause diarrhea.

All supplements are not dangerous or foolish, of course. You may well need to take extra calcium for your bones, and many studies show that women who take extra folic acid before they become pregnant and while they are pregnant are likelier to give birth to babies with normal brains and spinal cords than women who do not.

Here are my tips on "natural" products and supplements:

- It's important to check with your doctor, dietician, or other professional before beginning natural products or supplements. (Salespeople are not always reliable. I once inquired about a bin of pennyroyal in a natural foods and tea shop. The saleswoman told me how restorative it is. I said, "Did you know that pennyroyal has been used for centuries to cause abortions?" "No," she said.)
- The Internet is most helpful when the authority for a web site is the United States government, a respected research

institution, or a data-based not-for-profit; *http://medlineplus. gov* is a splendid resource for well-written information on a wide range of health and medical topics.

- Headlines are supposed to grab your attention so you'll buy the magazine or wait through the ads on TV or radio. They don't claim to educate or tell the truth.

- Bone up on science. Research is not a collection of anecdotes made popular by the herd mentality. Rather, good research meets high standards of ethics and reproducibility.

- Valid studies, depending on their purpose, generally enroll large numbers of people (more than 10-100) and continue for a long time (more than 6-12 months).

- Valid studies have a "control group"—some people receive the treatment and others don't. In "double-blind" tests, neither the researchers nor the subjects know which group is getting the medicine and which is getting the placebo. This precaution takes into account the fact the people have a remarkable propensity to feel better or worse even if they have a placebo.

- Valid studies report side effects and adverse outcomes along with efficacy. This includes reports on diets.

To add a further cautionary note, a product or supplement that is "natural" may act like a drug. Dr. Douglas Paauw, Professor of Medicine at the University of Washington School of Medicine, collects data on interactions of herbs and supplements with over-the-counter and prescription medication. These interactions are usually discovered by accident when humans are unwitting and unwilling experimental animals. Dr. Paauw cites a long list of "g" substances that interact with warfarin (Coumadin), an oral agent that is used to inhibit blood clotting:

- Garlic
- Ginger
- Ginseng
- Ginko
- Glucosamine/chondroitin
- Feverfew and dong quai (the latter is often used for gynecologic complaints without quality control or proof that claims are substantiated)

Similarly, St. John's wort, which has been used with inconsistent results for depression, has variable formulations of flowers, leaves, and/or stems. It interacts with statins and warfarin.

There is no room for guesswork with any herbs, or over-the-counter or prescription drugs. Tell your doctor absolutely everything that you eat or drink so he or she can determine what potential you have for negative interactions. The information you give your clinician needs to include alcohol consumption. Alcohol interacts with a host of medications, including some for allergies, infections, arthritis, cough, depression, high blood pressure, pain, sleep, and of course, warfarin. Some over-the-counter drugs contain a surprising amount of alcohol: Nyquil Cold and Flu is 10% alcohol. Compare that to beer (4% alcohol) and wine (11.5% – 15% alcohol). Full disclosure heightens your chance of avoiding a nasty herb, supplement, over-the-counter, or prescription interaction.

Restful Sleep

Nearly all of us experience sleeplessness at some time during our lives. Half of us have trouble sleeping more often than once a week. That can spell trouble, since the value of sleep is profound.

Sleep improves resilience, memory, insight, creative thinking, attention span, reaction time, and your ability to recover from fatigue. Thomas Edison may have invented the light bulb on three hours of sleep per night, but your lights are likely to dim with fewer than seven to eight hours.

Sadly, if you are weary, you often sleep fitfully. Your sleep is strained, even agitated, as your brain churns. This has got to stop. The Fatigue Prescription has some ways and means.

You know some old-but-good keys to restful sleep: no caffeine after noon (its effects can last twenty-four hours), cope with worries during daylight, and get your exercise well before bedtime. What else can you do to capture what Shakespeare called "Nature's soft nurse"?

One thing you should *not* do is rely on so-called "sleep aids"—namely, prescription or over-the-counter sleeping pills. I have one word to describe these drugs: dangerous. In a version of the Supplement Syndrome, there is a high risk of over-medicating yourself, as in "Gee, I slept pretty well on a single one of those; maybe I'll try two tonight." There is also risk of becoming dependent on these drugs. Then there is the danger of combining medications with each other, or with sedatives such as alcohol. Finally, if you use drugs to avoid dealing with the basic problems that may be keeping you awake, this is a recipe for disaster.

My advice: do not take sleep-aid drugs except in a real emergency. Even then, use only a prescription written by a reliable physician, and use it only for a night or two.

What about melatonin, the so-called "natural" sleep aid that is today's stylish preventative for jet lag? The same dangers apply. Plus, research has not shown the appropriate dose. We don't know melatonin's short-term or long-term effects; we don't know much about its interactions with other substances. In short, melatonin has not been well-studied and I think it can put your brain in jeopardy. That makes it too dangerous to mess with.

There may be reasons why you can't sleep. Maybe arthritis is producing a dull but persistent pain. If you're a woman in menopause or a man taking hormones for prostate cancer, you may have night sweats. Maybe you have regular, low-level headaches and you think if you could just ease the pain, you'd get a good night's sleep, and the headaches would be gone for good. Can't you just take a pill for it?

Maybe, but even the simplest remedies have side-effects. Aspirin can cause bleeding; other non-steroidal anti-inflammatory drugs, such as ibuprofen (Advil and Motrin) and naproxen (Aleve) can damage your kidneys; acetaminophen can cause liver failure. (Tylenol is one trade name; it is also found in Midol, Vicodin, Percocet, and some versions of Nyquil and Dayquil) These medications should be taken rarely and with restraint, even under a doctor's care. You should not take more than 4,000 milligrams of acetaminophen—and probably less—per twenty-four-hour period *alone or in combinations*. That means if you take a couple of acetaminophen-containing painkillers or sleep aids at night—which could be more than a gram—you are limiting the amount of the medication during the day.

There is no such thing as a secret formula or magic bullet to help you sleep, but I do have some recommendations.

- Open a window or turn the air conditioner on low; most people sleep better in a cool room.
- Tune in to some calming music, white noise, or nature sounds.
- An occasional relaxing bath or hot shower can help you put a *diminuendo* to the day.
- After the soak, you might choose some light reading material that takes your mind somewhere else, somewhere pleasant or amusing. That leaves out suspense and mayhem novels.

- If you think a nightcap will help, how about warm milk? It works. Alcohol can rev you up before it knocks you out.
- Think of your bed as, well, a bed. It is not an office, waiting room, library, storage closet, or cafeteria. A bed is for sex and sleep. You want just to look at your bed and think: make love or go to sleep. *Not* make a phone call; browse a magazine; have a snack.
- Is there a TV you can watch from bed? Get rid of it. News or talk-show hosts are not conducive to pleasant rest. Nor is listening to a police scanner. Get rid of the glowing clock, too. You can get agitated just eyeing it at night when you check to see what time it is and how long you've been asleep—or awake.
- Find something lovely to visualize. I often choose a peachy sunset over the ocean. After a trip to Hawaii and a long encounter with sea turtles, I see them with my mind's eye, suspended in the crystal clear green water, peaceful and utterly at home, and it usually puts me right to peaceful sleep.
- As for that low-level pain you may be tempted to assuage with a pill or two, try a gentle hot-water bottle instead. This antique remedy can soothe pain and provide sweet comfort. Electric heating pads can overheat or spark a fire. I do not recommend them.
- Always remember the cuddle, kiss, pats, and words of love as you drift off.

It takes awhile for fatigue to recede. One woman at a RENEW workshop said, "It took a year for me to get creative after I finally started getting enough sleep. It was like a veil lifting."

Take a Break

On any adventure, you need to take breaks.

Breaks can be short or long. A shrewd nurse once told me that the only way she could get off the unit during her shift was to go to the bathroom, so she drank a lot of water while she was on duty. For longer breaks, you could emulate the astute ministers, physicians, teachers, and executives who arrange for sabbaticals. You might be able to get funding from outside your organization to take a learning or service break. Some foundations are so concerned about the sustainability of the non-profit sector and its leaders, for example, that they offer grants to provide respite from the inexorable pressures.

At RENEW sessions, we often ask about micro-breaks: "What can you do in fifteen seconds to have a better day?" Here are some of the answers people frequently give.

MICRO-BREAKS	
Smile.	Wash your hands, splash your face.
Laugh!	Hold the elevator for someone.
Hug someone.	Put your head down on your desk.
Pet the dog; stroke the cat.	Think of someone you love.
Take a big, deep breath.	Kiss.
Smell a flower.	Pray.
Say "No."	Count your blessings.
Say "Yes."	Recall a pleasant memory.
Have a daydream.	Thank someone.

MICRO-BREAKS	
Stretch.	Take off your shoes.
Close your eyes.	Open your window, or at least look out of it.
Look at a favorite photo.	Exercise, even just five jumping jacks.
Send an xoxoxo text message.	Turn off the "received email" beep.

WHAT BREAKS CAN YOU TAKE?
My fifteen-second quick fixes:
What I could do with a longer break:
Very long breaks that I will schedule:

YOU'VE GOT ATTITUDE

We all have attitude, whether we know it or not, and we show it in the way we carry ourselves and interact with the world. And I'm sure it will come as no surprise when I tell you that a negative attitude, one of anger, fear, or annoyance, is exhausting. Clenching your teeth in fury or cowering in terror, whether literally or figuratively, are sure paths to fatigue.

So how can you fix your attitude and reduce your fatigue? Four things: get clear on what you can and cannot control, think well of yourself, have a sense of humor, and know how to be happier.

Control

The urge to control is virtually universal among high-reaching people. Unfortunately, it is damaging and wearing—both for you and for those around you. I've seen people with serious fatigue who have severe muscle pain as a direct result of the muscle-tensing that comes from trying to grasp and mold all their priorities. In fact, health consequences of fatigue range from widespread aches to nighttime teeth-grinding to increased blood pressure, all associated with tensions, frustrations, and explosions.

Our minister, Pam Shortridge, says: "We grasp for power and control when we are afraid." This is a good time to practice managing those urges to control and to fix. The Fatigue Prescription will give you the ability to let go of the things you should let go of.

I learned about control late, but well. As my parents' health was failing, I pulled out all the stops to reverse the trend. When they declined inexorably, however, my goals slowly shifted from "control" to "manage," then to "influence" and then, as Dr. Elizabeth Kübler-Ross called it, to "death with dignity." Along the way, I learned that I couldn't fix that which I wanted the most to fix, my beloved parents' health.

In our RENEWing workshops around the country, we ask, "What can you control?" Here are some answers:

THINGS I CAN CONTROL	
My aspirations	What I want to learn
The dog (sometimes)	The food I eat
What I put in my environment	The clothes I wear
My priorities and my actions	My attitude
What I worry about	My mood
Who I spend time with	My reactions
Information flow	How fast I drive
My mouth	What I do in my free time
My clutter	What I read
The way I treat others	My hair color
My decisions	How I spend my money
Sleep, to a certain extent	

Notice this list tends to omit the illusion (or delusion) of controlling other people or circumstances.

But for the sake of brevity, let's distill this list. The three most important things you can control are:

- *Your aspirations.* This implies going beyond hopes and dreams and into action.
- *Your behavior.* What you say and how you say it; what you do and when you do it.

- *Your attitude.* Because somehow the world tends to act the way you expect it to act. Or it becomes what you perceive it to be, the old self-fulfilling prophecy.

The Fatigue Prescription is all about giving you control over what you can control. It is about managing your energy, health, and life.

Self-Esteem

Your self-esteem is one of your best renewable energy sources. It can propel you over hurdles of fatigue and on to living your dreams. To "buff up" your self-esteem, you need to get some insights into why it may need burnishing and why it is essential to controlling your fatigue. Then you can develop ways to shine in your own light.

Why do you give yourself such short shrift sometimes? Or often? Perhaps you think you aren't worth the trouble? You may feel inadequate and unworthy. Why? Your self-esteem bucket may not have been filled early in life, or it may have been drawn down over time. Perhaps you are trying to be perfect and you can't be, so you are disappointed in yourself. If you've given up on perfection, you may still feel that it is your fault when things go wrong.

What is so splendid about self-esteem? Like it or not, you are the one upon whom you can most depend. You need to know you can do the job! Self-worth gives you the confidence to move forward. You need to have a good supply of pragmatic self-esteem to carry on in the face of opposition or disaster.

So let's fill your worthiness bucket. If you really examine yourself, you will find that you are quite fine. You are not a Nobel Laureate, perhaps, but you are far better than merely "acceptable." You have plenty of successes to celebrate, whether big or small. That means that you can reinforce yourself; you can refill your own bucket. I compliment myself every so often when I clear out a jumbled drawer, make points with students, or go for my (nearly) daily walk. "Way to go," I smile to myself when I weed the garden or put the spices in alphabetical order on the shelf. Give yourself plentiful compliments; this will raise your self-esteem.

Since part of gaining or regaining self-esteem also depends on how others see you, look in the mirror before you go out. A fashion consultant once said, "You are treated the way you look." Jamie wears a sport jacket and slacks on most airplane trips, and he notices that he receives better treatment from security officers, gate personnel, and flight attendants.

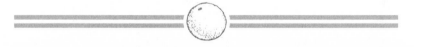

MY SELF-ESTEEM BUCKET
1. Level of self-esteem: ❑ High (watch out for overconfidence) ❑ Sufficient   ❑ Endangered   ❑ Low   ❑ Fumes
2. List three things you are good at:
3. My bucket needs attention and this is what I will do to fill it:

A Sense of Humor

Laughter changes everything, including your attitude. Losing your sense of humor is both a serious warning of dangerous fatigue and a loss of one of your major defense mechanisms. Laughter can help with embarrassment, enhance social relations, diffuse awkward situations, and, most of all, keep you happy.

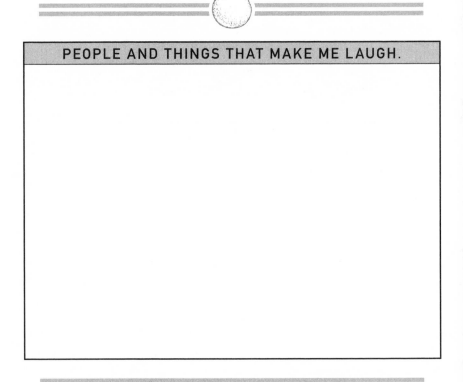

PEOPLE AND THINGS THAT MAKE ME LAUGH.

Your chuckles and guffaws set your own tone. Just hearing yourself laugh raises your spirits and the spirits of those around you. By enhancing your energy and health, laughter can fire you up as you uproot fatigue.

Happiness

Insofar as it is a choice, happiness is an attitude. Happiness—enjoying life, finding joy, and having fun—is right up there on the values popularity list with love. Happiness applies to the Fatigue Prescription in two ways: it is a way to quell fatigue, and it is a by-product of quelling fatigue.

I do recognize that some cynics scoff at the thought that happiness is possible or desirable. They say that if you are happy, you just don't get it—that you are a social and political blockhead.

Surely no one feels that life is or should be perpetual jubilation. Everyone keens and moans at times. That's Life. How would you know when you achieve the glow of happiness if you hadn't seen the dark side? But how does "enjoying life" actually feel? Can you achieve it these ragged days? If so, how?

Medical literature suggests that those who consider themselves happy may have longer and more productive lives. Vaillant cites a study of nuns, for example, that linked happiness and health. At age twenty, 180 nuns wrote a short autobiography. "Of those who expressed the most positive emotion, only 24% had died by age 80. In contrast, by the same age, 54% of those who expressed the least positive emotion had died."

So, happiness is good and it is something you have some control over. How can you get more of it?

The Dalai Lama, who is emphatic about good spirits, suggests that we are all seeking better things in our lives, seeing this as a movement towards happiness. A practice this wise man advises is to identify what leads to suffering, eliminate this from daily life, and spend time in the cultivation and pursuit of happiness.

MY OWN HAPPINESS

My definition of happiness:

What makes me feel peaceful or content?

What/who makes my heart warm?

What/who really excites me?

What/who makes me smile?

RENEWING RITUALS

Rituals fit into the Fatigue Prescription because they provide pattern and structure. Rituals also support and enhance your core—reflecting, connecting, and living your values and meaning. This section will define and describe some healthy rituals, what they do, and how to set them up.

Rituals can be practical. When I was an intern, I appreciated the routines we had for doing various punctures, drainages, and biopsies. They covered every part of the procedure from start to finish. They gave me confidence because if I followed them precisely, they were pretty foolproof, even for someone who was sleep deprived.

Rituals can also have a rich, dreamlike quality about them. Rituals offer opportunities to be in touch with your life force and its creativity, insights, and resilience. They are more than habits. They connect you to your essential self and remind you that you matter. Rituals can heal.

Rituals are likely to be everyday matters, except for the ones you hope are once-in-a-lifetime, such as a wedding. Some daily "ceremonies" may happen in the early morning—a cuddle, a latte, listening to NPR, a quiet time. They may happen in the evening—kids' bath time, reading, knitting, connecting, reflecting. On a more than daily basis, Jamie and I kiss each other and say, "I love you" every time we come home or leave home.

I have been surprised at the variety of practices that people consider "rituals." There are common threads among them: repetition, noticing, pondering, enjoying, and taking time. Here are some renewing rituals:

- Running or walking
- Going to church or synagogue
- Gardening, watering

- Saying grace at dinner
- Doing stretches in the shower
- Greeting the sunrise and acknowledging the new day
- Lighting candles at mealtime
- Walking the dog
- Writing
- Morning coffee

For people who are driven to produce and accomplish, these rituals may seem frivolous. I believe, however, that grinding on without relief wears us out. Rituals provide a renewing break. They can erase conflicts and fears and help inspiration seep in.

Reflect about things that revive you. What are your rituals? Think of quickies, such as a morning stretch, or more languid ones, like settling into your armchair at the end of the day with your feet up and a good mystery in hand.

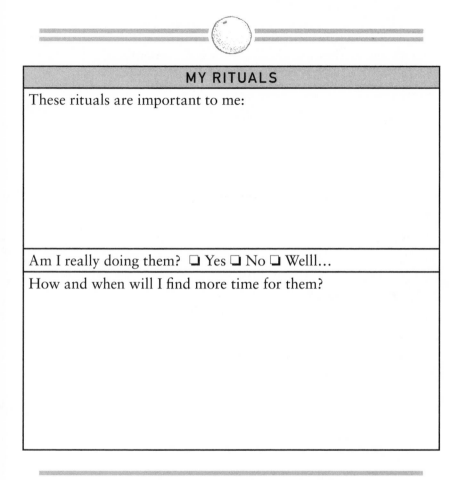

MY RITUALS

These rituals are important to me:

Am I really doing them? ❏ Yes ❏ No ❏ Welll...

How and when will I find more time for them?

The workout never really ends. As a personal trainer might say, you can always do one more repetition. Set your own buff-ness plans for fighting fatigue. And don't forget: you can't get buff overnight. This adventure is for the rest of your life.

As writer Henry Miller said, "One's destination is never a place, but a new way of seeing things." Fortunately, renewing is a splendid adventure. The Greek poet, Cavafy, who lived in

Alexandria, Egypt, imagined Odysseus' life as the great warrior struggled to get home to Ithaca after the Trojan Wars.

ITHACA

When you start on your journey to Ithaca,
then pray that the road is long,
full of adventure, full of knowledge.
Do not fear the Lestrygonians
and the Cyclopes and the angry Poseidon.
You will never meet such as these on your path,
if your thoughts remain lofty,
if a fine emotion touches your body and your spirit.
You will never meet the Lestrygonians,
the Cyclopes and the fierce Poseidon,
if you do not carry them within your soul,
if your soul does not raise them up before you.

Then pray that the road is long.
That the summer mornings are many,
that you will enter ports seen for the first time
with such pleasure, with such joy!
Stop at Phoenician markets,
and purchase fine merchandise,
mother-of-pearl and corals, amber and ebony,
and pleasurable perfumes of all kinds,
buy as many pleasurable perfumes as you can;
visit hosts of Egyptian cities,
to learn from those who have knowledge.

Always keep Ithaca fixed in your mind,
to arrive there is your ultimate goal.
But do not hurry the voyage at all.
It is better to let it last for long years;
and even to anchor at the isle when you are old,
rich with all that you have gained on the way,
not expecting that Ithaca will offer you riches.

Ithaca has given you the beautiful voyage.
Without her you would never have taken the road.
But she has nothing more to give you.

And if you find her poor, Ithaca has not defrauded you.
With the great wisdom you have gained, with so much
    experience,
you must surely have understood by then what Ithaca means.

(Translated by Rae Dalven)

CHAPTER 8

LIBERATED FROM FATIGUE AND STAYING RENEWED

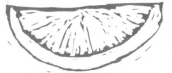

"If the odds weigh against...[filling] your days with joy...take a moment to ponder life's cosmic odds and how you've already beaten them."
—Reverend Forrest Church

Because it is not a one-off event, the Fatigue Prescription needs periodic boosts. Part of the pick-me-up is to keep in practice with the prescription itself. In this chapter, I will offer a quick quiz on the four steps—awareness → reflection → conversation → and plan-and-act—as it applies to your family as well as to yourself. Also, because you will need to make sound decisions and to face those lurking perils—fear, anger, and procrastination—I'll supply a few plans for doing so. Hanging on to your lifelines and remembering your values, even when they change, will also be in your curriculum. I have added a short discussion of time and having a positive perspective to the agenda to help you. You can also learn priceless ways to say, "No" so you don't skid into fatigue again. At the end, I will proffer some summary pointers on staying *up*.

From this altitude, you can see where you have been and where you are going. By now, you have considered your meaning and purpose, assayed your talents and put together your team, developed strategies, and drafted tactics. These are huge steps. Take a break to celebrate! Put gold stars on pages you love in this book. Leap for joy. Go to a karaoke joint. You are ready to launch.

THE FATIGUE PRESCRIPTION AS A FAMILY MATTER

As you can tell, I believe that family and friends are an integral part of a fulfilling, fatigue-free life. To me, "family" can be biological or preferential. I maintain that families and friends are examples—good or bad—and there's plenty to learn from them. They are more likely to be there for you than colleagues or strangers are. They can be the source of fun, sweetness, strength, and comfort. A family can help you dump fatigue.

Consider these statements about your family's health:

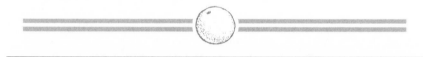

MY FAMILY'S HEALTH AS A FAMILY
The adults have confidence in each other and enjoy each other. We sort through differences and back each other up. ❏ Yes ❏ No
Across generations, we are open and kind with each other. We listen carefully, tell the truth, and laugh a fair amount. ❏ Yes ❏ No
We are independent yet respectful and like to learn from our tiffs. ❏ Yes ❏ No
We follow our family's rules. ❏ Yes ❏ No

MY FAMILY'S HEALTH AS A FAMILY

We do things together at least weekly (meals, performances, volunteering, practicing our faith, play). Or, because we live far apart, we enjoy touching base via phone or social networking. ❏ Yes ❏ No

---

MAKING GOOD CHOICES

Staying on top means making good decisions. This section provides ten guideposts to keep you on track.

1. *Have your values in mind.* For example, are your decisions kind and respectful? Are they healthy? Do they conform to your other important values?
2. *Have your goals and purpose in mind.* This includes reassessing them all the time to make sure you're still working toward what you want to be.
3. *Gather as much data as possible* to fortify your confidence. What are the financial and emotional costs of the decision? What have others learned from trying this?
4. *Estimate your and others' ability and readiness to take on the challenge.* This could affect your timing and direction.
5. *Plan to replenish yourself.* Schedule refreshers and rest stops to fill your energy bucket. Have good repair people—friends, advisors, Encouragers—around to help with this.
6. *Discuss the choices with important people* in your life. Be willing to change your mind.
7. *Acknowledge your fears,* including your fear of going up the wrong mountain. The side trips and discoveries could even be the start of something greater. Detours can become main thoroughfares.

8. *Build up your courage, curiosity, and resilience.* This will help you be ready for anything.
9. *Make a list* of positives and negatives and weigh them carefully.
10. *Consult your gut.* In our data-driven society, intuition often gets ignored. It is based on experience and wisdom, however, and is valuable.

CONTENDING WITH FEAR, ANGER AND PROCRASTINATION

You can count on fear being at the edges or the center of a new venture, but fear isn't all bad. It can activate you. Gavin de Becker discussed ways to avoid violence in his book, *The Gift of Fear.* He gave examples of people in peril who paid attention to signals and instincts, contrasted with people who did not. Outcomes were far better for those who registered fear and acted upon it.

How can you best handle fear? One of my walking companions, therapist Joan Schretlen, points out that people can choose how they want to act, even in the most desperate circumstances. She offers the following pointers:

MANAGING FEAR
Acknowledge your fear.
Accept your fear. Embrace the unknown and know that the "right" thing will happen.
You have choices about how to handle fear. Losing control is voluntary.
Keep putting one foot in front of the other, no matter how frightened you are. If you give in to fear, it multiplies.
Try some self-hypnosis. Find an image of peace and tranquility, a place that connects you with the world. Put yourself in that place and take ten deep slow breaths. Relax and repeat to yourself, "Everything is going to be fine" or "I can do this."

Another approach to managing fear, even the kind that may linger, is to ask, "What would I do if I were not afraid?" If I weren't afraid of failing, might I take that exciting job at the start-up? If I weren't afraid of getting put down, might I suggest my sensational idea? If I weren't afraid of looking funny, would I take that hula course that seems like so much fun? Naming fears—and recognizing choices—can help you gain the nerve to press on. It is the same with anger.

Anger seems to feed on itself and spread. It not only causes a cycle of distress within you, but it spills onto others. A taxi driver once told me that he had finally figured out that his brother had used angry outbursts to manipulate his family for years. Everyone tiptoed around him, avoiding anything that would unleash the brother's rages. After the cabbie's "Aha!" moment, the family decided to give up kowtowing; the torrents of anger no longer swamped their good humor and plans.

This is a good time to visit your shadow lands.

MY FEAR AND ANGER
What am I afraid of?
What am I angry about?
Are my feelings interfering with me or others? ❏ Yes ❏ No ❏ Not quite yet
How will I start to grapple with them?

Procrastination is an all too common strategy used by many, including perfectionists (like me and maybe you). Many of us have this foot-dragging art form, well, perfected. A historically thorough social worker told me, "If you ever see me rearranging my recipe file, you know that I should be doing something more important."

Sometimes you don't start or finish projects because you want to get them *right* at the cost of getting them *done*—or at the cost of going home on time, making decisions, or taking care of yourself. Delaying tactics can also be used just because you don't want to do something or because you dread it.

Procrastination does not have to rule you. Here are two of the best ways to resist its dominion:

1. Look forward to the reward and be sure to give yourself one.

2. Don't do the hard things first.

The advice about rewarding yourself is pretty straight-forward. Getting work done is a pleasure in itself—and even better if you take five and have some fun afterwards. Delaying gratification wears out faster for your family and friends than for you, but even you feel tired and cheated after days or years of putting off pleasure.

"Don't do the hard things first" is counter-intuitive if you like the high fives and the glory of moving in fast for the score. The problem is, not many Hail Mary passes win the Super Bowl. Games are won mainly by slogging along, making first downs in several plays.

There are several beauties to starting easy.

For one, if the hard problem could have been solved before, it probably *would* have been solved before. You may be in over your head from the get-go. In addition, a small project—raising funds to buy a few children's books for the library—has a high likelihood of turning out well. First off, you learn what doesn't work, in private, and you can correct it. Those who work together can enjoy the flush of accomplishment. Building a team and building a community begin. As a sense of effectiveness grows, others want to join in and the way clears for the next, perhaps bigger, undertaking. Putting pieces of a puzzle together one by one, even with some mistakes along the way, builds a whole new library, rebuilds an inner city, or reunites a family.

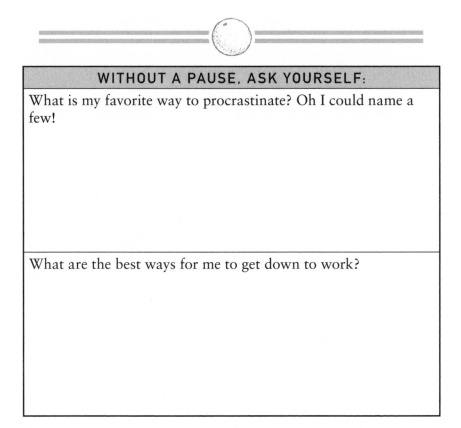

WITHOUT A PAUSE, ASK YOURSELF:

What is my favorite way to procrastinate? Oh I could name a few!

What are the best ways for me to get down to work?

Sometimes hard things must be done first. You don't have the luxury of procrastination when a family member has an accident. Even if your preference is to delay, knowing your values and purpose gets you going, pronto, and the Fatigue Prescription has paid off.

UPDATING YOUR VALUES

As I have mentioned, values are essential anchors. Yet your experiences may transform your outlook and the territory itself may alter. Here is a list of some "renovations" in fundamentals that I have heard. Values didn't disappear; they got remodeled.

- People are becoming more important than accomplishments. Maybe that's because I've lost some dear people.
- I see myself as important, not just my work. I decide what is truly necessary to do so that there is more "me" left at the end of the day.
- I'm not delaying gratification as much, so I'm living in the moment, trying to bloom where I'm planted. I'm taking better care of myself.
- I am even more determined to improve the world, but now I see that my lifetime is limited.
- I'm increasing my reliance on others.
- I want to have more fun, do more traveling, and help others more.
- I've become concerned about the environment, and the importance and fragility of communities.
- I've chosen to become more optimistic. I've also given up some arrogance and taken on more humility.

In Chapter 5, you examined how your values have developed and evolved. As you have put the Fatigue Prescription into play, do you want or need to revamp your values at this point? In what way?

MAKING TIME

The Greeks have several words for time. *Chronos*, the root of *chronology*, refers to the actual passage of time—minutes, days, seasons in sequence. *Kairos* means time in the sense of the "right" or "opportune" time. *Schole* means leisure time or spare time, a time to collect your thoughts.

You may feel trapped in *chronos*. The Fatigue Prescription suggests lengthening *chronos* with *kairos* and *schole*. Because remember, you can't tell quality time with a watch.

Making time is hard, but it's necessary and worth it. I bet you've heard or said, "I don't want to miss my child's childhood." Children do grow fast and move away. One way to help them boomerang back is to make good memories by spending time together.

On our family outings, I used to be the planner. But I got tired of making arrangements about the same time that Jamie and Sarah got tired of getting dragged around according to my whims. We found that we made better memories—spent better quality time—when we alternated the responsibility (and pleasure) of planning our days. So we would go to a restaurant that had waiters on roller skates, and then go to art exhibits, too.

Some people with hectic schedules have made good time in other ways. One social worker covers the pages of a calendar with favorite quotations and poems upon which to reflect. A CEO commented that he literally puts time slots in his days for thinking. And you? What have you done lately to make time for reflection, for conversation, for fun?

MAINTAINING A POSITIVE PERSPECTIVE

Within limits, you can choose your outlook. Plenty of good things happen every day, and an upbeat outlook helps them happen more often.

My Great Auntie Verle used to say whenever I got in a dither, "If that's the worst thing that ever happens to you, it isn't very bad." I had enough imagination to snap out of it. You aren't in a tent in Pakistan or homeless in New Orleans. Listening to others' predicaments is another way to get a grip on reality. There is almost always someone else worse off than you. A woman I know talked herself out of the blues by using comparisons, "We have to move into a smaller house. We just can't afford the big one anymore. But at least we have a house."

It has been shown that a positive perspective leads to higher spirits. Researchers note that even elders with several disabilities are happier than predicted, perhaps because their lives had prepared them to be pragmatic. I love these anecdotes:

- When he was eighty-one, Henry Jones, Emeritus Professor of Radiology at Stanford observed, "I'm feeling just great. Of course, if I had felt this way when I was seventeen, I would have called 911."
- Surgeon Leonard Rosenman, also eighty-one, said, "I'm perfect. At my age, 'perfect' is three things: when you wake up in the morning, you realize you can breathe. When you open your eyes, you realize you can see. And only two things hurt."
- Stanford Professor Hernat Katchadourian noted, "I'm doing very well, considering my highly reduced expectation."

It is true that bad things happen and being positive doesn't erase them. The idea is to acknowledge the negatives, grieve, and then shift gears and move forward, out of fatigue.

STAYING IN TOUCH WITH YOUR LIFELINES

Lifelines keep you from drifting off course. They intercede with a gentle or sharp tug, which can even save your life. They are part of your lifelong equipment to avoid fatigue and stay renewed. Who are your lifelines? Yourself. Others you are close to. Your principles. Your protectors. Your Encouragers. Keep in touch with these people and things, which can see you through the toughest times.

You Are Your Own Lifeline
In Chapter 1, you itemized your signs of trouble. You might want to see how you are measuring up now. You could also compare yourself with a group of not-for-profit leaders who met a couple of years ago to renew. Early on, they talked about being aware of their danger signals. Do you recognize any of yours in this list?

DANGER SIGNALS	
Sleep too much	Don't sleep well
Blame others	Become indecisive
Get negative	Can't see solutions
Get less curious	Lose hope
Have less sense of humor	Don't ask for help
Snap at others	Feel defensive
Curse	Breathe differently
Can't focus	Have irregular bowel movements
Become non-productive	Drink alcohol
Forget	Wake up exhausted
Isolate	Eat too much
Make enemies from allies	Become lethargic
Have constant anxiety	

In the "connecting with me" department, you can also check out where you are in relation to all the things you have to do. Are you getting help when you need it? Are you making time for things that matter?

AM I DOING MY TO-DO'S?
1. How is my calendar? Any time for thinking, frolicking, taking care? ❏ Some ❏ Good trend ❏ Slipping
2. Am I doing my must-dos, including connecting with others? ❏ Yes ❏ No Here are some I'm doing
3. Am I learning things? ❏ Yes ❏ No If yes, what
4. What have I delegated—and to whom?
5. Have I asked for help if I needed it? ❏ Yes ❏ No If no, why not? If yes, how is it going?

While connecting with yourself, you can't really avoid your body. In Chapters 2 and 7, you profiled your health and your health maintenance. If it's time for a new fitness routine, consult Chapter 6 for a refresher on the nuts and bolts of change and your own barriers and boosters to change. No body, no mission!

Sustaining Friendships

Pooh and Piglet are an example of an enriching friendship that many of us read about at an early age. In a conversation about the first thing that each says upon waking, Pooh asks himself, "What's for breakfast?" Piglet wonders "What's going to happen exciting today?" Pooh sagely recognizes that Piglet's answer is the same as his own.

Good company, Pooh and Piglet. You need good company, too—good friends and family. They are the webbing that helps keep you together. They are key to filling and refilling the Fatigue Prescription. After all, "conversation" is step three and you have conversations with others, mainly.

How can you sustain friendships? How about sending notes (in ink, not only email) and flowers? Or taking and sharing photos? You can let your special people know in big and small ways that they are in your heart. I sent cards to my high school teacher Dorothy Volgenau for decades. She offered me an unforgettable bit of advice with a twinkle: "Linda, don't ever tell a lie. You're just terrible at it."

You can never say thank you enough to your dearest ones—or anyone. We thank our son-in-law Keith Gayler for the books and notes he sends us even when it isn't a birthday or Christmas. We thank him for his wizard technology skills, movie and gallery reviews, and brave, sweet temperament. I also appreciate his basic principles, one of which is, "My starting point is that people want to help you. I remember what it's like to have been helped and I enjoy helping others in return." I especially thank him in my mind for those sentiments when I'm starting a conversation with a ticket agent or customer service representative. I thank Jamie, too, for all of the little things—and the big thing of putting up with me in general.

What else can you do to keep friendships fresh? You can adjust your life. One physician said, "I took a decreased salary to increase my free time. I coach soccer. So what if our cars are older? I took a cut to three-quarters time and three-quarters pay but I still get full benefits. It's a win-win."

People at RENEW conferences have further ideas:

- We may eat late, but we eat together. We have discussions about feelings at the table. We don't just rehearse the plots of TV shows.
- We swim together.
- We take a kid-less twenty-four hour break every six months to talk about our successes and problems.
- I don't take any work home. The job is a bottomless pit. If I do take something home, I put it in the den, far away from everyone else so it doesn't contaminate us. I get my reading done in half hour snatches during lunchtime at work.

Sometimes, to keep family and friends close, you have to take a stand. A real estate attorney said, "I was letting my clients push me around. I needed the business but I was not being my own master. One Christmas time, a broker called me eight or nine times a day. He was nasty. My kids were begging for my time, but he kept yammering. I finally told him that I wanted to spend time with my kids and my kids wanted to be with me and this whole thing was interfering with my life. He said, 'I get it. Okay, I won't call until after the New Year.' The deal closed January 14."

Take a moment and think of ways you link with family and friends and how you manage to get together: potlucks, music, bowling, shopping until you drop.

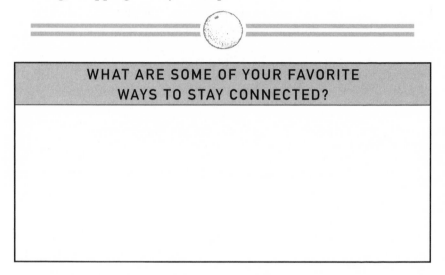

WHAT ARE SOME OF YOUR FAVORITE
WAYS TO STAY CONNECTED?

Remembering Values
For most of us, life is way too short for frustrating mazes and exhaustion. To keep myself on the straight and narrow, I decided that I needed a simple way to remember my values. I came up with my "F" list. It is a strange, mixed lot that is incomplete but I wrote down and say aloud, to help the principles stick in my brain even when I approach warp speed.

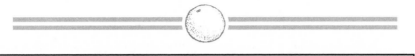

LINDA CLEVER'S "F" VALUES
Family
Friends
Faith
Flexibility
Fun
Fear
Fight
Freedom
Chocolate*

*Actually, Fudge

I listed "fear" not because I like it but because it can be a compelling force for change. I included "fight" because sometimes you have to summon your courage and stand up for your beliefs. "Freedom" is on my list because it is so important to me and others—such as the freedom to wear what you wish or marry whom you love. Chocolate (or fudge) stands on its own.

Jamie has a "C" list:

JAMIE CLEVER'S "C" VALUES
Courage
Community
Connection
Creativity
Clarity
Cooperation
Commitment

Now it's your turn! How will you prompt yourself about values so that you don't have to spend any time thinking about them? The more explicit your values are, the more they are a part of you, and the easier they are to activate when you need them.

Once you've got your list clear and sure, you can decide how to keep yourself in touch with it. Will you put your values on your key chain or bracelet? Or your screen-saver or rearview-mirror dangling doodad? Or in a list, haiku, prayer, or song?

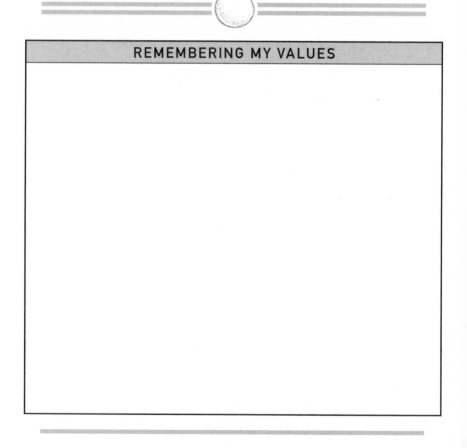

REMEMBERING MY VALUES

SAYING NO—AND YES—AT THE RIGHT TIME

You probably already know that fatigue stems from overdoing it, whether over-extending or over-committing. The effects of fatigue are as toxic as any other overdose and can be just as permanent. It is therefore smart to stop fatigue before it starts. One way to head it off at the pass is to say no more often. This section will give you some idea about why you say yes and why you don't say no. It will show the advantages of saying no and how to reverse the yes trend.

Why You Do Say Yes When You Should Say No?

Just as I said at the beginning of Chapter 1 about the genesis of your fatigue, your yeses and nos are shaped by the way your nature, nurture, and circumstances intertwine. Your main impetus may be that you want to accomplish important things or keep up with the flood of obligations. You may be afraid of letting someone down or letting something go. Or you may be pretty convinced that you can do something better than anyone else. You may be building a career and want to prove yourself. You certainly don't want to look weak, or be considered a shirker. You may like praise or the spotlight. Or maybe yes is merely an ingrained habit. Any and all of these can lead you to say yes when you really ought to say no.

The Perks of Saying No

"No" is a way of showing respect for whoever is asking you to take on a commitment or project. Think about it: If you become wearied from fatigue, scheduled to the max, overburdened, and oversubscribed, how much value can you really add to the next thing you are asked to do—even if the next thing sounds appealing? The likely answer is less than you suppose and less than is needed.

Saying no is also a way of keeping healthy for the long run. Humans weren't made to be in perpetual motion. The *quality* of your activities matters, not the *quantity*. Saying no to a double shift could save you from falling asleep at the wheel and totaling the car on your way home from work. Saying no to the next tight deadline may give you time to go to the gym or take a walk—and come back rarin' to go because of the energy lift. Saying no to the next community initiative, worthy though it may be, may allow for a family or solo vacation, which could prove even more nurturing to body, mind, and soul—and replenish your passion for the cause and your ingenuity for solving problems. There is no way around it. There are limits to what you can do, and there are limits to what you *should* do in order to stay fit and functioning.

Perhaps most importantly, saying no to pressure from others is a way of saying yes to yourself. It is proof of your self-esteem. It says, "I will take care of myself and my aspirations. I will not let others sap my energy or my time. I will live my values and accomplish my priorities. I will not undermine my health. Because *I matter*."

Bottom line? Saying no can be good for you in many ways.

Take a second to think about some things you wish you had said no to. It may not be too late to change them, and even if it is, this will help you avoid doing the same thing next time.

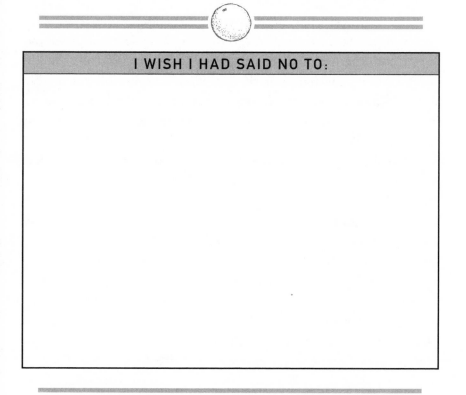

I WISH I HAD SAID NO TO:

How to Say No

You won't faint when I suggest that you start to say no more often when you review your values. That shouldn't be so hard, now that you have them plastered all over your house, car, office, and mind. In that context, ask yourself whether all of your yeses are entirely congruent with what matters most to you. If not, here are some ways to get back on track:

- *Delegate:* Ask someone else to take something over at home, community, or work.
- *Creative destruction:* Identify what can go and let go of it.

- *Versioning:* Have Version I, then Version II and III, and so forth. Clarify the scope and the life cycle of each version and then move on to the next.
- *Review your goals and accomplishments:* Maybe you've already done what you set out to do.
- *Get new ideas* from outside the committee or the institution.

It is better to say no in the first place, of course, since prevention is better than treatment. William Ury, in *The Power of a Positive No: How to Say No and Still Get to Yes*, posits that a "Positive No" is the "crux of the process, requiring skill and tact. It begins with an affirmation (*Yes!*), proceeds to establish a limit *(No)*, and ends with a proposal (*Yes?*)." I call this the "No Sandwich."

It takes forethought to prepare a good No Sandwich. So if you're going to go to that trouble, you have to be sure it's worth it. Invoke the Twenty-Four-Hour Rule (ask for a day to consider the offer) so you can check your values again and see if the proposal fits with all of them. This short time-out might also let you see that you don't have the energy to do well whatever is being asked right now. Maybe by getting someone else involved, the organization could get a better result. This works at home, too, although it may take some effort to find alternatives or stand-ins. Also, you realize that saying no doesn't mean giving up. It means grabbing the opportunity to take a breather and recover from fatigue. There is nothing wrong with that. As I noted earlier, if you're too tired to do justice to what you've been asked to do, what's the point of doing it?

For the legions of us who have a hard time saying no, savvy "No" practitioners offer some successful principles and phrases. These are the meat of the No Sandwich. The first layer of the Sandwich is admiration (of the task) and thanks (for the honor of being asked). Then comes the meat, and then the last layer is offering other options (if you wish) and thanks. Here is the meat, the part of the No Sandwich that actually says no:

- *Defer:* "I'd love to do it, but you deserve and need a better job than I can do right now."
- *Give compliments:* "This is important work, but it is not my work."
- *Don't complain, don't explain.* Just say "No" or "No, thanks."
- *Give the "No" a little humor:* "This is my year for saying no."
- *Set limits:* "I'm getting behind on work right now. I can't do anything else and do it well."
- *Point out the facts:* "My plate is full. I have no room for anything else."

If you don't want to say a firm no but are willing to offer options, you could try the following:

- *Offer a trade:* "I'll need to take something else off my plate. I could do this if I don't do that."
- *Suggest a possible deferral:* "I cannot do this now, but maybe later."
- *Get advice:* "How do you suggest I get this all done?"
- *Mention helpers:* "Can anyone else pitch in?"

When you experiment with saying no to family and friends, at work, or in your neighborhood, keep track of what happens. How did you feel at the time? Later? What did the asker say and do? What were the consequences, negative and positive? Decide whether, next time, you should try the same approach or a different one. Using the No Sandwich—at the right time, in the right way—saves energy and builds stamina.

STAYING UP

We have worked hard and well, you and I, with the Fatigue Prescription. It's an adventure, all right, getting rid of fatigue and staying renewed. I hope you have reached a high point using the four steps, and I hope you like being at or near the mountaintop.

We will all have downs. I hope your work with the Prescription will provide extra resilience. It is meant to be like a trampoline. I find a sign that Sarah gave me very reassuring: POBODY'S NERFECT. That takes a good deal of pressure off; it helps with getting the bounce back.

In a capsule, here are a few things I want you to be sure of:

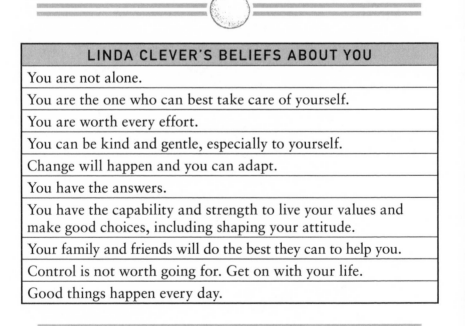

LINDA CLEVER'S BELIEFS ABOUT YOU
You are not alone.
You are the one who can best take care of yourself.
You are worth every effort.
You can be kind and gentle, especially to yourself.
Change will happen and you can adapt.
You have the answers.
You have the capability and strength to live your values and make good choices, including shaping your attitude.
Your family and friends will do the best they can to help you.
Control is not worth going for. Get on with your life.
Good things happen every day.

Because you never know when your trajectory will move from up to down, it's important to have an abundance of good memories, good will, and energy to help you cope. I have developed a philosophy I call "moderated hedonism": live it up but don't hurt yourself or anyone else; life is too short for regrets.

Now that you have the four steps of *The Fatigue Prescription*— awareness → reflection → conversation → plan-and-act—all squared away, you could use your re-filled energy bucket to make your own bucket list. You really don't want to be like my friend's aunt, who bought a brand new pink dress but was saving it for a big occasion. The right occasion never came along, and they buried her in the dress with its price tag still on.

MY WILL-DO LIST
What matters most to you? List as many answers as you like.

With your fatigue gone, you can do it all—just not all at once. Remember, "moderated hedonism."

Good, fatigue-free health to you!

AFTERWORD

Grab this book and take a ride on the Renewal Railroad, jettisoning unneeded life baggage on the way to a more energized, stress-free, and meaningful future. The good doctor gives us a prescription in detail for self-renewal, complete with humor, stories, wisdom, and worksheets. Read it, learn, laugh, and write yourself to a more energized life.

It's about you. It's about renewal. It's about living, loving, learning, and putting it all together in a better way so you can enjoy and savor as well as contribute and challenge yourself. Give yourself a gift. Read the book and then pick up your pencil and work through the exercises. You will emerge uplifted.

Linda Hawes Clever writes as she speaks—with humor and content abundant. We are lucky to have this book to keep at hand, to revisit her wisdom, to work through the challenges, and to keep as a reference as we move forward from fatigue to full power. It is a unique contribution to all who are committed and tired as well.

Francesca Gardner
Editor of *Living, Leading, and the American Dream*

RESOURCES

INTERNET

Health

Centers for Disease Control
Prevention and control of disease, injury, and disability; preparedness against new health threats. Includes infections, vaccines, and mysterious epidemics.
www.cdc.gov

Mayo Clinic
Medical information and tools for healthy living.
www.mayoclinic.com/health/HealthyLivingIndex/HealthyLivingIndex

Medline Plus
Well written and authoritative general health and medical information for the public.
medlineplus.gov

National Heart, Lung and Blood Institute
Promotes the prevention and treatment of heart, lung, and blood diseases.
www.nhlbi.nih.gov

National Institute on Alcohol Abuse and Alcoholism
Conducts and supports research in a wide range of scientific areas, including genetics, neuroscience, epidemiology, health risks, and

benefits of alcohol consumption, prevention, and treatment.
www.niaaa.nih.gov

National Institute on Drug Abuse
Research and information on drug abuse and addiction.
www.nida.nih.gov

National Osteoporosis Foundation
Voluntary health organization devoted to osteoporosis and bone health.
www.nof.org

Office of Dietary Supplements of the National Institutes of Health
Evaluates and disseminates scientific information; stimulates and supports research, and educates the public about dietary supplements.
ods.od.nih.gov

PubMed
Access to original scientific papers and abstracts via the National Library of Medicine of the National Institutes of Health.
www.pubmed.gov

Vaccination Information
Vaccine information for the public and health professionals.
www.vaccineinformation.org

Quotations

quotegarden.com
quoteland.com

www.brainyhistory.com/quotes
www.quotationspage.com
thinkexist.com/quotes
www.dailygood.org
www.charityfocus.org/new
www.wisdomquotes.com
www.thetao.info

Reports

"Growing Older in America: The Health & Retirement Study." National Institute on Aging, U.S. National Institutes of Health, www.nia.nih.gov/ResearchInformation/ExtramuralPrograms/BehavioralAndSocialResearch/HRS.htm.

"Retirement at the Tipping Point: The Year That Changed Everything: New Fears, New Hopes, and a New Purpose for Retirement." Age Wave, www.agewave.com/RetirementTippingPoint.pdf.

"Your Guide to Physical Activity and Your Heart," U.S. Department of Health & Human Services, www.nhlbi.nih.gov/health/public/heart/obesity/phy_active.pdf.

PUBLICATIONS

Books

Babcock, L. and S. Laschever. *Women Don't Ask: Negotiation and the Gender Divide.* Princeton University Press, Princeton, 2003.

Bracken, P. *The I Hate To Cookbook.* Harcourt Brace & Company, New York, 1960.

Bridges, W. *Managing Transitions: Making The Most of Change.* Perseus Books, Redding, MA, 1991.

Bynner, W. *The Way of Life According to Lao Tzu.* Putnam Publishing Group, New York, 1994.

Church, F. *My Journey Through the Valley of the Shadow.* Beacon Press, Boston, 2008. Reprinted in *Stanford Magazine* (Nov./Dec.) 2008: 62-64

Cialdini, R.B. *Yes!: 50 Scientifically Proven Ways to Be Persuasive.* Free Press, New York, 2008.

Collins, J. and J. Porras. *Built To Last: Successful Habits Of Visionary Companies.* Harper Business Essentials, New York, 1997.

Covey, S.R. *The Seven Habits of Highly Effective People: Powerful Learning In Personal Change.* Simon Schuster, New York, 1989 (15th Anniversary Version, 2004).

Csikszentmihalyi, M. *Flow: The Psychology of Optimal Experience.* Harper & Row, New York, 1990.

Dalai Lama and H.C. Cutler. *The Art of Happiness: A Handbook for Living.* Riverhead Books, New York, 1998.

de Becker, G. *The Gift of Fear.* Dell Publishing, a division of Bantam Doubleday Dell Publishing Group, Inc., New York, 1997.

Evans, G. *Play Like A Man, Win Like A Woman: What Men Know About Success That Women Need To Learn*. Broadway Books, New York, 2000.

Fisher, R., and W. Ury. *Getting to Yes: Negotiating Agreement without Giving In*. Houghton Mifflin, Boston, 1981.

Freeman, C. *Wisdom Made in America*. Walnut Grove Press, 1995.

Gardner, J.W. *Excellence: Can We Be Equal and Excellent Too?* W. W. Norton & Company, New York, 1995.

Gardner, J.W. *Self Renewal: The Individual and the Innovative Society, Revised Edition*. W.W. Norton & Company, New York, 1995.

Gibran, K. *The Prophet*. Alfred A. Knopf, New York, 2002.

Goleman, D., Boyatzis, R., and A. McKee. *Primal Leadership: Realizing the Power of Emotional Intelligence*. Harvard Business School Press, Boston, 2002.

Goleman, D. *Emotional Intelligence*. Bantam Books, New York, 1995.

Hammond, S.A. *The Thin Book of Appreciative Inquiry, Second Edition*. Thin Book Publishing Company, Plano, Texas, 1998.

Herbert, G. *The Poetical Works of George Herbert*. Caswell, Petter & Galpin, London, 1875.

Johnson, S. *Who Moved My Cheese?* G.P. Putnam's Sons, New York, 1998.

Kabat-Zinn, J. *Arriving at Your Own Door: 108 Lessons in Mindfulness*. Hyperion Books, New York, 2002.

Lundin, S.C., Paul, H. and J. Christensen. *Fish!* Hyperion, New York, 2000.

Magee, M. *The Book of Choices: A Treasury of Insights for Personal and Professional Growth*. Spencer Books, New York, 2002.

Murray, W.H. *The Scottish Himalayan Expedition.* J.M. Dent & Sons, London, 1951.

O'Neil, J.R. *The Paradox of Success: When Winning At Work Means Losing At Life.* Putnam Publishing Group, New York, 1994.

Palmer, P.J. *Let Your Life Speak: Listening for the Voice of Vocation.* Jossey-Bass, San Francisco, 2000.

Remen, R.N. *My Grandfather's Blessings.* Riverhead Books, New York, 2000.

Rubin, L. *The Transcendent Child: Tales of Triumph Over the Past.* Harper Paperbacks, New York, 1997.

Ury, W. *The Power of a Positive No: How to Say No and Still Get to Yes.* Harper Collins, New York, 2007.

White, E.B. *Charlotte's Web.* HarperTrophy, New York. Original copyright 1952, renewed in 1980.

Zeldin, T. *Conversation.* Harvill Press, London, 1998.

Journal References

Bickel, J. and A.J. Brown. "Generation X: Implications for Faculty Recruitment and Development in Academic Health Centers." *Academic Medicine* 80 (2005): #3.

Boyle, P.A,. Barnes, L.L., Buchman, A.S., and D.A. Bennett. "Purpose in Life Is Associated with Mortality Among Community-Dwelling Older Persons." *Psychosomatic Medicine* (71) 2008: 574-579.

Gardner, J.W. "Personal Renewal." *Western Journal of Medicine* 157 (1992): 457-459.

Giltay, E.J., et al. "Dispositional Optimism and All-Cause and Cardiovascular Mortality in a Prospective Cohort of Elderly

Dutch Men and Women." *Archives of General Psychiatry* 61 (2004): 1126-35, reported by N.L. Stotland, in Journal Watch Women's Health 10 (2005):15.

Johnson, S. "Organizing Your Work and Time." *Academic Physician and Scientist* September (2004):2-3.

Kaufman, D.M. "Applying Educational Theory in Practice." *British Medical Journal* 326 (2003):213-216.

Maruta, T., Colligan, R., Malinchoc, M., and K. Offord. "Optimism-Pessimism Assessed in the 1960's: Self-reported Health Status 30 Years Later." *Mayo Clinic Proceedings* 77 (2002):748-753.

Morowitz. H.J. "Optimism as a Moral Imperative." *Hospital Practice* February (1983): 237.

Sherman, B. and N. Quinn. "Using Stages of Change to Motivate Patients." *Clinical Care Update* 8 (2002):1-2.

Vaillant, G. E. "Mental Health." *American Journal of Psychiatry* 160 (2003): 1380.

Zimmerman, G.L., Olsen, C.G., and M.F. Bosworth. "A 'Stages of Change' Approach to Helping Patients Change Behavior." *American Family Physician* 61 (2000):1409-1416.

Journals of General Interest

Annals of Internal Medicine
British Medical Journal
Journal of General Internal Medicine
New England Journal of Medicine

Newsletter Reference

U.C. Berkeley. *Wellness Letter: The Newsletter of Nutrition, Fitness, And Self-Care* 20 (Feb. 2004): 1.

Newsletters of General Interest

Harvard Wellness Letter
Journal Watch

ABOUT RENEW

RENEW is not just a word or a concept. RENEW is a movement.

My friends, colleagues, and I started RENEW, a not-for-profit organization, in 1998 with inspiration from John W. Gardner. It is a special project of the Institute for Health and Healing at San Francisco's California Pacific Medical Center.

RENEW aims to help busy, devoted people sustain or regain enthusiasm, effectiveness, meaning, and, yes, joy. We believe that people have deep reservoirs of talent, wisdom, and courage. We also see that people who live their values have remarkable energy and purpose. Therefore, recognizing and refreshing personal values are both key to accomplishing high goals.

The ability to RENEW requires reflection, practice, and feedback. This means that RENEWing takes some quiet time. Interactions, encouragement, and a robust sense of humor all help.

RENEW offers several ways to restore creativity, resilience, and relationships. We give presentations (including keynotes), workshops, consultations, seminars, and a series of remarkable RENEWing Groups. We also teach people how to convene

RENEWing Groups. RENEW's activities follow a similar pattern. They are planned jointly with institutions, organizations, and businesses so that they meet the groups' wants and needs. More participation than presentation, sessions focus on sound, feasible information with strong underpinnings and proven results. They acknowledge the interweaving of body, mind (intellect and emotions), and spirit. We have a good time too, as people connect and move forward.

In addition to living your values, RENEW emphasizes several things, such as the intersections and conflicts of work and personal life; barriers and boosters to change; leadership; courage; "homework" with family, friends, and colleagues; and communication.

Does RENEWing work? People say that it builds team collaboration and effectiveness and fosters good practices during changes and crises. We hear about innovative problem solving, newly flexible thinking, and individuals who regain capability and peace. We see re-fueled empathy and whole, healthy lives.

RENEW helps people live their values with good health. We figure: if you stop learning and stop changing, you stop living.

Visit RENEW online at www.renewnow.org.

ABOUT THE AUTHOR

Linda Hawes Clever, MD, MACP, is founding President of RENEW, a not-for-profit aimed at helping devoted people maintain (and regain) enthusiasm, effectiveness, and purpose. She is also a member of the Institute of Medicine of the National Academy of Sciences, Adjunct Clinical Professor of Medicine at Stanford, Clinical Professor of Medicine at UCSF, former Editor of the *Western Journal of Medicine*, and founding chair of the Department of Occupational Health at California Pacific Medical Center.

Dr. Clever received undergraduate and medical degrees from Stanford University and had several years of medical residency and fellowships at Stanford and UCSF in internal medicine, infectious diseases, community medicine, and occupational medicine. Dr. Clever was the first Medical Director of the teaching clinic at St. Mary's Hospital in San Francisco where she started patient education and nurse practitioner training and research programs. She started the Department of Occupational Health at the then-Pacific Medical Center and began her activities in the American College of Physicians in which she served as Governor, Chair of the Board of Governors, and Regent. She has written numerous papers, chapters, articles, and editorials. Her areas of special interest include personal and organizational renewal; intersections of life, work, and health; the occupational health of women and heath care workers and leadership.

She served on the Stanford University Board of Trustees for fourteen years and has chaired the Boards of KQED and University High School. She now serves on the Board of the Northern California Presbyterian Homes and Services and chairs its Foundation Board. Her husband Jamie is also an internist as is their daughter Sarah, who is on the faculty of the Johns Hopkins School of Medicine. Dr. Clever likes walks, good conversations, and good cookies.